MANUAL OF HAND SPLINTING

Nancy M. Cannon, O.T.R.

Rebecca W. Foltz, O.T.R.
Jan M. Koepfer, O.T.R.
Melanie F. Lauck, O.T.R.
Dawn M. Simpson, O.T.R.
Roberta S. Bromley, O.T.R.

The Hand Rehabilitation Center of Indiana, Inc.
Indianapolis, Indiana

Churchill Livingstone
New York, Edinburgh, London, and Melbourne 1985

Acquisitions editor: Kim Loretucci
Copy editor: Ann Ruzycka
Production editor: Karen Goldsmith Montanez
Production supervisor: Joseph Sita
Compositor: Maryland Composition Company, Inc.
Printer/Binder: The Maple-Vail Book Manufacturing Group

1198/213

Distributed in the United Kingdom by Churchill Livingstone,
Robert Stevenson House, 1–3 Baxter's Place, Leith Walk,
Edinburgh EH1 3AF and associated companies, branches
and representatives throughout the world.

First published in 1985

Printed in the U.S.A.

ISBN 0–443–08451–3

9 8 7 6 5 4 3 2 1

Library of Congress Cataloging in Publication Data

Main entry under title:

Manual of hand splinting.

   Bibliography: p.
   1. Hand—Wounds and injuries—Treatment. 2. Splints
(Surgery) I. Cannon, Nancy M. [DNLM: 1. Hand Injuries—
therapy. 2. Splints. WE 830 M294]
RD559.M28 1985   617'.575044   85-6664
ISBN 0-443-08451-3

Manufactured in the United States of America

In dedication to

James W. Strickland, M.D.
James B. Steichen, M.D.
William B. Kleinman, M.D.
Hill Hastings II, M.D.
Richard S. Idler, M.D.

who, in their unending contributions to the realm of hand surgery, have inspired and supported us in this endeavor.

PREFACE

The *Manual of Hand Splinting* has been written as a general, introductory guide for the physician and therapist involved with the management of basic upper extremity problems. The manual's purpose is to show the reader the more commonly used splints and indicate practical applications for those splints.

The Introduction reviews the basic anatomical and biomechanical considerations with upper extremity splinting. In addition, many of the types of commonly available splinting products on the market today are reviewed.

The nomenclature for hand splinting is discussed. The reader should realize the splinting terminology in this manual is a system which the authors have developed through the years with a group of hand surgeons. Since the naming of splints is currently not standardized, a physician and therapist must work together to develop a common splinting terminology. At some point in the future we should see a more standardized nomenclature for splinting.

Photographs have been used throughout the manual to clearly illustrate the appearance of the splints on the hand. The angle selected for each photograph provides a view that should enable most therapists to fabricate many of these splints by the photograph alone. With some of the more complex splints, a detailed description of how to fabricate the splint is provided.

The information presented with each splint provides the reader with an overview of the type of splint, the splint's purpose, the indications for using such a splint, suggested wearing times, correct fit, and precautions.

The goal in developing this manual was to combine and condense many years of experience in hand splinting into a valuable guide which is readily accessible and easy to interpret. The authors hope the manual meets your needs and achieves this goal.

Nancy M. Cannon, O.T.R.
Rebecca W. Foltz, O.T.R.
Jan M. Koepfer, O.T.R.
Melanie F. Lauck, O.T.R.
Dawn M. Simpson, O.T.R.
Roberta S. Bromley, O.T.R.

ACKNOWLEDGMENTS

The authors would like to acknowledge the following individuals for their professional skills used in developing this splinting manual: Cathy Fazio and Gary Schnitz, medical illustrations and photography; Maureen Sanner, photography; Jo Ann Hildebrand and Lori Bagal, typing. Additionally, the authors would like to acknowledge the work of Karan Harmon-Gettle, O.T.R., Indianapolis, Indiana, for initial work in preparing splinting handouts at The Hand Rehabilitation Center of Indiana, Inc. It is from that initial format that this splinting manual developed.

TABLE OF CONTENTS

ABBREVIATIONS

A	Active	ORIF	Open reduction internal fixation
AA	Active assistive	P	Passive
CMC	Carpometacarpal joint	PIP	Proximal interphalangeal joint
DBS	Dorsal blocking splint	PRN	As needed
DIP	Distal interphalangeal joint	P_1	Proximal phalanx
ECRL	Extensor carpi radialis longus	P_2	Middle phalanx
EDC	Extensor digitorum communis	P_3	Distal phalanx
FCR	Flexor carpi radialis	RA	Rheumatoid arthritis
FCU	Flexor carpi ulnaris	RCL	Radial collateral ligament
FDP	Flexor digitorum profundus	RN	Radial nerve
FDS	Flexor digitorum superficialis	ROM	Range of motion
FPL	Flexor pollicis longus	SBRN	Superficial branch radial nerve
IP	Interphalangeal joint	UCL	Ulnar collateral ligament
MN	Median nerve	UN	Ulnar nerve

MANUAL OF HAND SPLINTING

INTRODUCTION 1

He who works with his hands is a laborer,
He who works with his hands and his mind is a craftsman,
He who works with his hands and his mind and his heart is an artist.

Author unknown

Due to the supreme need for optimal hand function in human activities, rehabilitation following an injury is paramount.

Splints act as a means for delicately controlling, preserving, modifying, and affecting motion so that the desired end result is more likely to be achieved.

This manual clearly demonstrates the need for a strong knowledge of anatomy biomechanics of the hand, and of diagnoses and surgical management in order to splint the hand properly.

TYPES OF SPLINTS

Splints may be classified as custom-made or prefabricated and may be either static or dynamic in function. Static splints prevent motion and are used to immobilize or stabilize in one specific position:

> For protection
> To rest joints
> To decrease inflammation and pain
> To prevent undesired motion
> To substitute for lost muscle function

Long periods of immobilization in static splints without the appropriate accompanying exercise program may lead to stiffness, weakness, and dependency. Therefore, when these splints are used, the patient's therapy program should include a balance of exercises and splinting to be maximally beneficial.

Dynamic splints permit the controlled movement of various joints. Their purpose is to apply traction in order to:

> Resolve tendon tightness
> Resolve fixed joint contractures
> Increase or maintain active and/or passive range of motion

When active range-of-motion exercises are not aggressive enough to overcome joint or tendon tightness, or when the joint is painful, gentle dynamic traction may resolve the problem.

Prefabricated splints are commercially available and generally come in several sizes. There are many varieties of these splints on the market and their number seems to be increasing. The physician or therapist choosing and applying a prefabricated splint must have a knowledge of the principles of mechanics and fit in order to use the splint appropriately and effectively. If the prefabricated splint does not fit well, it should not be used. A well-molded, custom-made splint should be designed and used instead.

NAMING SPLINTS

Splints are typically named by the function they serve or named by therapists in the various clinical settings. There is presently no standardized method for naming splints. However, the American Society of Hand Therapists has plans to establish a system of nomenclature for hand splinting. Until such a system is established, physicians and therapists must devise a system of nomenclature that they understand and interpret in the same way.

PARTS OF SPLINTS

In order to understand the names of various hand splints, the specific parts of the splints must be understood. The terminology used is not standardized, but is very com-

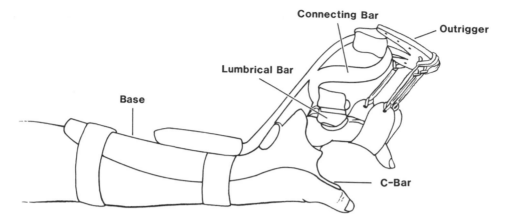

Fig. 1-1. Components of a long dorsal outrigger with lumbrical bar.

monly used among therapists. Figure 1-1 illustrates and identifies the basic components of a complex splint.

ANATOMICAL CONSIDERATIONS

Important features of hand anatomy must be respected with all types of hand-based splinting. The following are the primary areas to be taken into consideration.

Arches

The arches of the hand must be supported during splinting to preserve normal anatomical structures and provide comfort. The proximal transverse arch lies at the

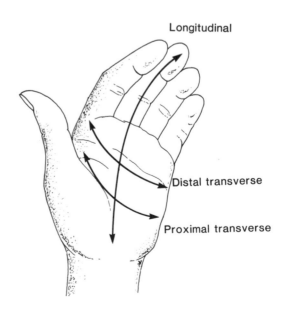

Fig. 1-2. Arches of the hand.

level of the distal carpus and is rigid, whereas the distal transverse arch passing through the metacarpal heads is more mobile. The transverse arches are connected by the longitudinal arch which consists of the second and third metacarpal, the index and long fingers distally, and the central carpus proximally (Fig. 1-2).

Creases
The distal palmar flexion crease is an important surface landmark. This crease must be totally cleared during splinting to allow full flexion of the metacarpophalangeal joints. Equally important are the thenar crease and finger creases, which are shown in Figure 1-3.

Bony Structures
Pressure must be avoided over bony prominences of the hand, wrist, and arm during splint fabrication. Problem areas include the metacarpophalangeal joints, the radial and ulnar styloid processes, the pisiform, the base of the first metacarpal, and the medial and lateral epicondyles. The splint must either clear these structures or allow sufficient space for them (Fig. 1-4).

SURFACE ANATOMY
(Volar surface)

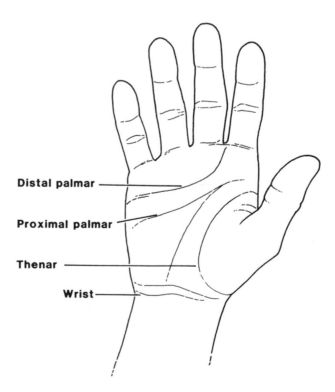

Fig. 1-3. Surface anatomy of the hand.

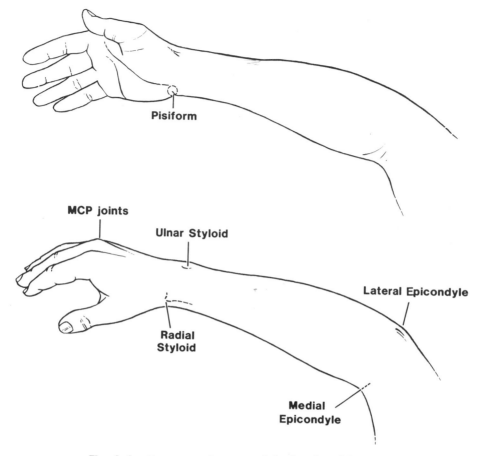

Fig. 1-4. Bony prominences of the hand and forearm.

Nerves

The superficial branch of the radial nerve (SBRN) is particularly vulnerable to compression during the application of a forearm-based splint. Forearm splints must not extend beyond the midlateral aspect of the forearm. If the radial edge of the forearm splint stops beyond the midlateral forearm, near the dorsum of the thumb, the superficial branch of the radial nerve may be compressed.

Ligamentous Structures

It is important to avoid ligamentous stress to joints during splinting. Lateral stress to joints, particularly with dynamic splinting, may cause unequal stretching of the collateral ligaments. In dynamic splinting, the traction must be applied perpendicular to the phalanx being mobilized. With static splinting similar consideration must be given to avoiding ligamentous stress. One example would be stretching the first web space during the construction of a web spacer splint. The ulnar collateral ligament of the thumb may easily be stressed as the therapist brings the thumb into radial or palmar abduction (Figs. 1-5, 1-6).

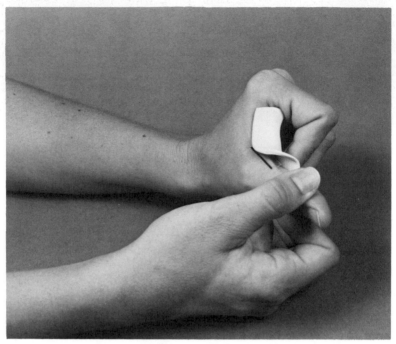

Fig. 1-5. Incorrect fit of web spacer splint causing stress to the thumb MP ulnar collateral ligament.

When dynamic traction is applied to the fingers the line of pull should be directed toward the scaphoid (Fig. 1-7). The rubber band traction for each digit should come from separate points of origin at the wrist level. By following these basic splinting principles, there is little chance of placing any undue stress on the digital collateral ligaments.

MECHANICAL PRINCIPLES

Mechanical principles provide the basis for the application of forces to the hand. Without an understanding of these principles, significant harm may be done to joint structures.

Angle of Pull

A 90° angle of pull from the outrigger to the phalanx being mobilized is essential (Fig. 1-8). When force is applied at an angle less than 90°, the sling transfers force to the articular cartilage. When the dynamic force is applied at an angle greater than 90°, the sling slips distally and causes distraction of the joint.

Dynamic traction to the wrist is applied at a 90° angle to the metacarpals. Attention should be given to ligamentous structures within the radiocarpal and midcarpal joints of the wrist since scar formation within various structures of the wrist may affect the application of dynamic traction (Fig. 1-9).

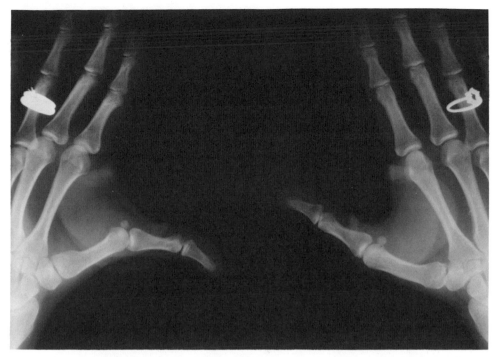

Fig. 1-6. (A) Radiograph to the left is demonstrating excessive stress being applied to the thumb MP joint ulnar collateral ligament during the construction of a web spacer splint. (B) Radiograph to the right shows minimal stress being applied to the collateral ligament with proper splint fabrication.

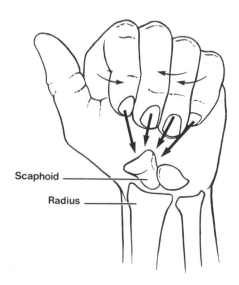

Scaphoid

Radius

Fig. 1-7. Dynamic flexion to the digits should be directed in the normal anatomical alignment toward the scaphoid.

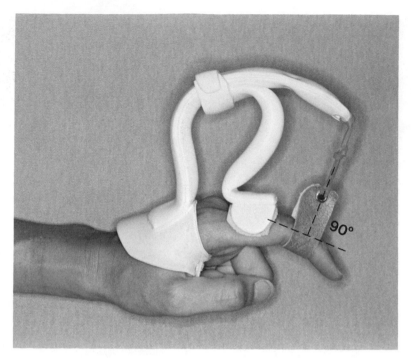

Fig. 1-8. With dynamic traction a 90° line of pull is essential to the bone being mobilized. The goal of this splint is to mobilize the middle phalanx in order to increase passive PIP joint extension.

Pressure

The formula:

$$\text{Pressure} = \frac{\text{total force}}{\text{area of force application}}$$

is particularly important in splinting. Each splint needs to be well-contoured and cover a large surface area to decrease pressure and prevent pressure sores on the hand. This same principle is important with splinting straps. The straps should be as wide as possible to distribute the pressure properly, and minimize localized edema.

Transfer of Pressure

Splints that cross the wrist should extend two-thirds the distance of the forearm. A longer forearm trough or lever arm decreases the resultant pressure caused by the proximally transferred weight of the hand to the volar forearm.

GENERAL PRINCIPLES OF FIT

Any splint should be comfortable, well-contoured by conforming to the longitudinal and transverse arches of the hand, simple to apply, stable on the hand, and cosmetically acceptable.

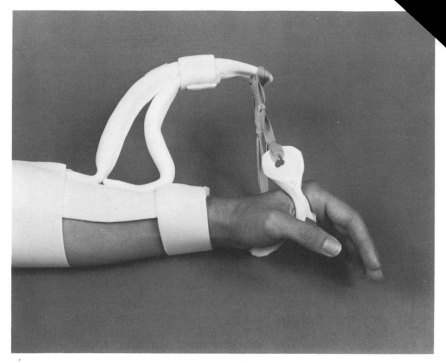

Fig. 1-9. Dynamic traction to the wrist is applied at a 90° angle to the metacarpals.

PRECAUTIONS

When splinting, one must consider potential problem areas and manage the splinting program accordingly. The primary areas to consider include pressure areas, edema, increased joint pain, and stiffness.

Pressure Areas

Patients with vascular insufficiency, sensory impairment, and thin tissue are especially prone to pressure areas from a hand-based splint. An improperly fitted splint may easily create such a problem for these individuals.

Vascular Insufficiency: The use of hand-based splints should be minimized in patients with a severely reduced vascular supply to the hand. Gradual skin breakdown will occur if pressure areas from a splint go unnoticed or uncorrected. The pressure area reduces the already impaired blood supply and nutrition to the area. The most appropriate splint for such a patient should have a large area of application and the widest possible straps.

Thin Tissue: Frequently the patient with rheumatoid arthritis has thin or fragile skin secondary to the medical management of the arthritis. For this reason, any arthritic splint must be well-molded to avoid bony prominences and prevent distal slippage of the splint across the skin. Patients with thin skin must inspect their skin daily to ensure that pressure areas are not being formed by the splints. If a pressure area does develop, simply padding the splint with moleskin or a foam material is not a valuable form of

the pressure area. Often a pressure area indicates that the splint
ig will only aggravate the problem. It is important to adjust the

hand with sensory impairment must be carefully splinted since
ating a potential problem are absent. Pressure areas may develop
s not frequently inspected by the patient and therapist.

Edema

Inflammatory edema occurs in varying degrees as a natural response to tissue damage; the compact structures of the hand are especially vulnerable to the presence of such fluid. Mechanical venous obstruction and dependent positioning of the hand are frequently cited factors which hasten the rate at which fluid transudes from the vessel to the interstitial spaces. Edema is increased in these cases. Intermittent elevation is a valuable means of reducing the edema.

The use of heat for edema control is the subject of controversy. The authors' experience has shown that heat has tended to increase edema in acute hand injuries. Therefore, the use of heat should be reserved until after the acute phase, if it is thought to be indicated.

When edema is significant (i.e., volumeter readings of 25 ml or greater than the opposite extremity) constricting splints must be avoided. Increasing the size of the area the splint covers and providing wide strap material are effective means of minimizing further swelling.

If a splint is being used to increase range of motion and the hand is edematous, the splint should be removed each hour for 10 to 15 minutes of active exercise. This improves circulation to the hand by allowing the intrinsic and extrinsic muscles to act as a pumping mechanism to the hand. Thus, arterial inflow and venous outflow are facilitated.

Effective measures to control edema include light compressive dressings, elastic bandage wraps, elasticized stockinette, Coban, "finger socks" sewn from elasticized bandage material, intermittent elevation, and the use of a snugly fitting surgical glove while exercising (Fig. 1-10). Resistive exercise should be avoided, since this will increase the already present edema.

SPLINTING MATERIALS

Thermoplastics

Most of the custom-made splints illustrated in this manual are made from low-temperature thermoplastics; these include Polyform, Orthoplast, Precision Splint, and Ultrasplint (Table 1-1).

The Polyform and Precision splint materials warm best by using wet heat such as water heated in a hydroculator or electric skillet. Orthoplast and Ultrasplint reach molding temperature with either wet or dry heat. Dry heat methods may include a heat gun or electric fry pan.

Each of these plastics reach molding temperature between 160 and 170° F within 1 minute. They may be cut with scissors and will harden within 3 to 4 minutes.

The low-temperature thermoplastics are very suitable for hand splinting as they can be worked with easily and quickly with a minimum of equipment. They conform well to the arches and contours of the hand and revisions may easily be made by heating the specific area of the splint that needs adjustment.

(Text continues on page 14.)

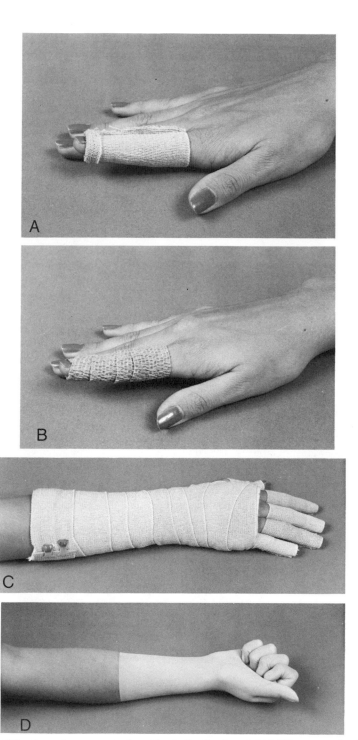

Fig. 1-10. Effective edema control methods for the hand, (A) "Finger socks." (B) Coban wrap. (C) Light compressive dressing. (D) Surgical glove.

Table 1-1. Comparison of Thermoplastic Splinting Materials

Trade Name	Properties	Positive Features
Aquaplast	Translucent, moderately rigid when hard. Totally transparent, sticky when soft. Available in two thicknesses (2 and 3 mm), three degrees of pliability, two perforation patterns, sheet sizes from 6" × 18" to 24" × 36".	Clings to contours during molding. Self-bonds without surface preparation. Returns to original shape when reheated. Color change indicates softening and hardening. Transparency allows for more exact placement of the splint, reveals potential pressure points.
Aquaplast T	Same as Aquaplast except not sticky and slightly cloudy when soft.	Advantages are similar to that of Aquaplast. Requires less skill to use.
Polyform and Kay Splint	Off-white opaque shiny surface. Nonelastic, puttylike, and very pliable when soft. Rigid when hard. Available in 3-mm thickness, smooth and perforated, in sheets of 18" × 24" and 24" × 36".	Exceptional rigidity and conformity. Bonds readily with surface preparation. Scraps can be reused. Pliability adjustable with water temperature.
Polyflex II and Kay Splint Isoprene	Same as Polyform except slightly less rigid when hard.	Greater temperature tolerance. Greater flexion tolerance.
Polyplast	Rigid and opaque when hard. Translucent, nonelastic, and waxy when soft. Available in 3-mm thickness, smooth and perforated, in sheets of 18" × 24" and 24" × 36".	Color change indicates softening and hardening. Edges finish easily. Pliability adjustable with water temperature. Scraps can be reused. Bonds readily with surface preparation.
Precision Splint (Similar to Kay Splint and Polyform)	Off-white shiny surface. Nonelastic, puttylike, and very moldable when soft. Very rigid when hard.	Exceptional rigidity and moldability. Moldability is adjustable with water temperature. Excellent self-bond when solvent is used. Scraps can be reused. Exceptional coating for smooth shiny surface. Material has a controlled stretch.

Table 1-1. (*Continued*)

Trade Name	Properties	Positive Features
Custom Splint (Similar to Polyflex) II and Kay Splint (Isoprene)	Subtle flesh tone color. Slightly less rigid than Precision Splint when hard.	Greater temperature and flexion tolerance than Precision Splint.
Sansplint and Orthoplast	Pink or stark white opaque matte surface. Semirigid when hard. Semipliable and elastic when soft. Available in 3-mm thickness, 18" × 24" and 24" × 36" sheets, smooth and perforated.	Requires least skill to use. Wide temperature tolerance. Bonds with surface preparation. Cosmetically appealing when new.
Ultra Splint (Similar to Orthoplast and E-Z Form)	A rubber-based compound. Unique feature is ability to restart a splint if a mistake is made. Material will return to its original cut shape when placed back into 160° water. The manufacturer claims better rigidity than other rubber-based compounds.	Excellent control when working with the material. Will retain its original cut shape when heated. Can activate a tackiness in the material when stretched to assist with self-adherence. Provides good conform-ability and drapability.
Kydex	High-temperature, rigid thermoplastic material. Material can be formed at 300–350°F.	Durable, retains good toughness even at sub-zero temperatures. Able to withstand repeated impact. Excellent when durability, toughness, and maximum rigidity needed.
Manorthos	Gleeming white surface. Puttylike molding properties with easy edge finishing. Lightweight and soil resistant.	Pliability may be adjusted to suit the splinting application. Excessive pliability can be avoided by minimal initial heating of the plastic with spot heating or reheating used where additional pliability is needed.

Information provided by Poly-Med Splint Company, Inc., Cockeysville, Maryland; and All Plastic, Inc., Indianapolis, Indiana.

With minimal surface preparation of the material, similar pieces of the plastics may be adhered to each other. This is advantageous because many splints require attachments such as outriggers to provide a point of origin for dynamic traction.

Kydex, a rigid high-temperature plastic, is often used as the outrigger on the long dorsal outrigger, certain short dorsal outrigger splints, and the dynamic splint for patients who have undergone silastic metacarpophalangeal joint arthroplasties. The outrigger pattern must be cut on a band saw or jigsaw and heated with a heat gun to contour. Three-eighth-inch Kydex is used. This material becomes pliable at 350 to 380° F.

Straps

The most common type of strap material used is Velcro. Adhesive-backed hook Velcro is used on the splint and the loop Velcro for the straps. Beta Pile, Duraval, and Velfoam are padded strap materials that may be used over sensitive areas. As mentioned previously, all straps should be cut as wide as is practical to decrease pressure.

Cuffs and Rubber Bands

Lightweight vinyl or leather cuffs with a cloth interfacing are used as slings to provide purchase on the proximal phalanx when the metacarpophalangeal joint is dynamically flexed or extended. Padded cuffs are occasionally used on patients with very sensitive or delicate skin.

Rubber bands used in hand splinting should be made of pure rubber, since these provide a more consistent dynamic pull. Number 32 (3 inches × ⅛ inch) rubber bands are usually used for most dynamic splints. The dynamic splint constructed for rheumatoid arthritic patients who have undergone silastic metacarpophalangeal (MP) joint arthroplasties uses number 18 rubber bands. This rubber band is 3 inches long and 1/16 inch wide and allows the patient to flex against the rubber band with greater ease.

Approximately 8 ounces of tension are generally used with the dynamic traction. The amount of tension on the rubber bands can be determined with a spring-type scale (Fig. 1-11).

When splinting acute hand problems, use slightly less tension with the dynamic traction. The likelihood of damaging the healing soft-tissue structures is greater in the acute phase and must be considered with all forms of dynamic as well as static splinting. In the case of MP arthroplasties, the dynamic traction should be less than 4 ounces of tension.

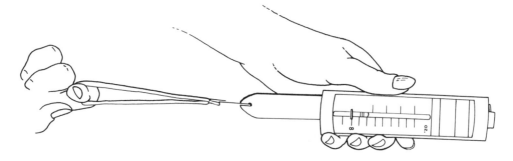

Fig. 1-11. A spring scale such as the one illustrated may be utilized to objectively establish the amount of tension being placed on a rubber band for dynamic traction.

MANUAL OF HAND SPLINTING

A newer product on the market for dynamic traction, referred to as "elastic thread," has also been shown to be an effective means of dynamic traction.

Outriggers

An outrigger is a point of origin for the application of dynamic traction and may be in the form of a ⅜ inch Kydex bar, an Orthoplast tube, or a piece of metal wiring arising from the base of the splint. The outrigger may extend from the splint base in a dorsal, volar, or lateral direction depending upon the purpose it is to serve.

The authors prefer the use of high-profile splinting to the low-profile approach, because it is much easier to adjust the splints. This prevents the need for fabricating new splints at frequent intervals and it is easier to determine if the dynamic traction is perpendicular to the bone being mobilized. This manual illustrates the high-profile splinting approach.

STATIC FINGER EXTENSION SPLINTS 2

MALLET FINGER SPLINT

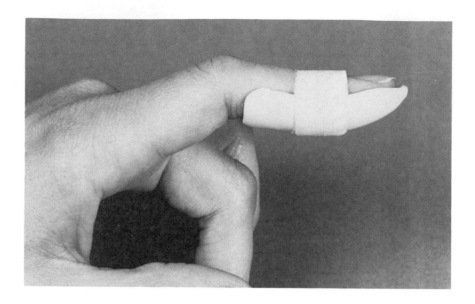

Type: Static

Purpose: To immobilize the DIP joint in slight hyperextension to approx-
                       imate a ruptured, lacerated, or avulsed terminal tendon of the
                       extensor mechanism

Indications: Rupture, laceration, or avulsion of the terminal extensor mech-
                       anism at the distal phalanx

Wearing Times: The splint is worn continuously except for cleaning.
                       Acute injuries (< 3 weeks from date of injury); the splint is worn
                       for 6 weeks.
                       Chronic injuries (> 3 weeks); the splint is worn continuously
                       for 8 weeks.

Precautions: The DIP joint must be held continually in extension even when
                       the splint is removed for cleaning.
                       Do not place a hypermobile DIP joint in more than 15° of hy-
                       perextension.

Correct Fit: Position DIP joint in slight hyperextension.
                       Place tape across the DIP joint for completion of the three-point
                       pressure.
                       Allow full range of motion of the PIP joint.

CYLINDER CAST

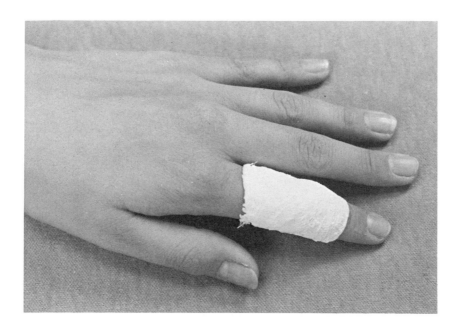

Type:	Static
Purpose:	To serially increase passive PIP joint extension (generally used with PIP joint flexion contractures less than 50°) To immobilize the PIP joint in full extension
Indications:	Soft-tissue injuries Arthrofibrosis secondary to trauma Boutonnière deformity P_1 and P_2 fractures (once clinically healed)
Wearing Times:	Generally worn at all times between exercises and at night. With boutonnière deformities, once the PIP joint is to 0° passively, it is held there for 6 to 8 weeks.
Precautions:	The patient should return for cast changes every 3 to 4 days. Watch for soft-tissue breakdown on the dorsum of the PIP joint. Edema may cause difficulty with removing the cast. Do not use before removal of sutures or with soft-tissue maceration.
Correct Fit:	The PIP joint should be held in full passive extension.

GUTTER SPLINT

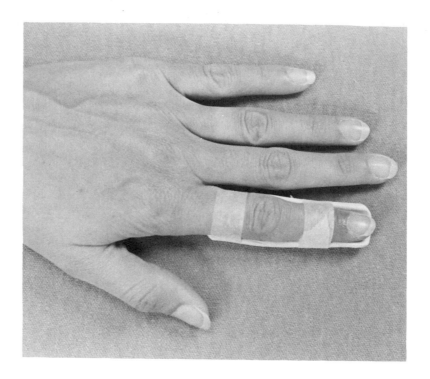

Type: Static

Purpose: To protect or immobilize the PIP and DIP joints in full extension

Indications: PIP arthroplasty
                     Boutonnière deformity (only the PIP joint is splinted)
                     Repair of digital extensor tendon
                     Extensor/flexor tenolysis
                     Fusion of the PIP or DIP joint
                     Phalangeal fractures (P_2 and distal P_1)

Wearing Times: Worn between exercise sessions following repair of the digital
                     extensor tendon. The splint is first applied at 4½ weeks post-
                     repair when AROM exercises are initiated and discontinued at
                     8 weeks.
                     Worn between exercise sessions to minimize extensor lags and
                     to protect from lateral stress following PIP joint arthroplasties
                     Worn between exercise sessions to prevent recurrence of a flex-
                     ion deformity following a PIP joint volar capsulotomy or flexor/
                     extensor tenolysis
                     Worn between exercise sessions to prevent extensor lags with
                     phalangeal fractures

Precautions: Watch for hyperextension of the splinted joints as well as lateral deviation.
Narrow straps may increase digital edema of the splinted joints.

Correct Fit: The gutter splint should position the indicated joints in full extension with the exception of fusions, which should be placed in their pinned position.
The gutter splint should have sufficient lateral height to prevent radial or ulnar deviation with PIP joint arthroplasties.
The straps of the gutter splint should rest proximal to the PIP joint and over the DIP joint.

TIP PROTECTOR SPLINT

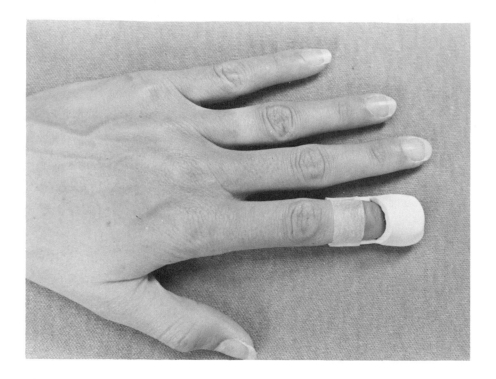

Type: Static

Purpose: To protect or immobilize the fingertip from external trauma

Indications: Digital amputations
                     Nail-bed injuries
                     Soft-tissue injuries
                     DIP joint pins from DIP fusion or mallet repair
                     Tuft fractures

Wearing Times: The tip protector is worn for protection during hand use and
                     may be removed to air the pin sites while the hand is at rest.

Precautions: The splint should not block motion to the PIP joint.
                     If the fit is too snug, it may cause discomfort at the pin sites.

Correct Fit: The splint should cover the distal phalanx, fit snugly around the
                     middle phalanx, and allow full ROM to the PIP joint.

FULL EXTENSION RESTING PAN SPLINT

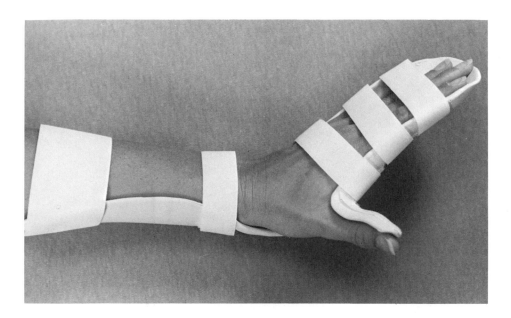

Type: Static

Purpose: To protect extensor tendon repairs and prevent extensor lags
To prevent or resolve extrinsic flexor tightness by gradually increasing wrist and digital extension
To maintain extension and prevent ulnar deviation following MP arthroplasties

Indications: Extensor tendon repairs (dorsum of the hand and forearm)
Volar MP and IP joint capsulotomies
MP joint arthroplasties
Flexor or extensor tendon tenolysis
Extrinsic flexor tightness (a minimum of 6 weeks post flexor tendon repair)

Wearing Times: Between exercises and at night following MP and IP joint volar capsulotomies and extensor tendon repairs
At night following MP arthroplasties.
Between exercises and at night following flexor and extensor tenolysis

Precautions: Prevent hyperextension of the MP joints by placing the MPs in 15° flexion.
Protect MP joint arthroplasties from hyperextension and ulnar deviation.

Correct Fit: The wrist should be positioned in 15° of dorsiflexion with the MP joints resting in slight flexion and the IP joints in full extension. In the case of extrinsic flexor tightness the wrist and digits should be positioned in maximum extension.

DUPUYTREN'S GUTTER SPLINT

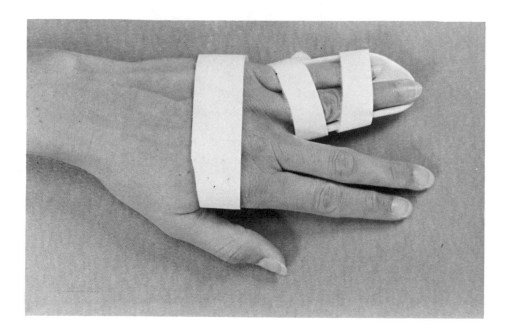

Type:	Static
Purpose:	To hold the MP, PIP, and DIP joints in full extension to prevent recurrence of a flexion deformity following a subtotal palmar fasciectomy
Indications:	Subtotal palmar fasciectomy
Wearing Times:	The gutter splint is worn between exercises and at night until extension is easily maintained. Once full extension is easily maintained (usually 6 weeks) the wearing time may be decreased to night only. The splint is worn at night for approximately 6 months.
Precautions:	Watch for hyperextension of the IP joints.
Correct Fit:	The MP, PIP, and DIP joints are held in full extension. The strap over the dorsum of the hand must be just proximal to the MP joint. The proximal portion of the gutter splint should rest just distal to the wrist to provide an excellent lever arm for MP joint extension.

DYNAMIC FINGER EXTENSION SPLINTS 3

BUNNELL SAFETY PIN SPLINT

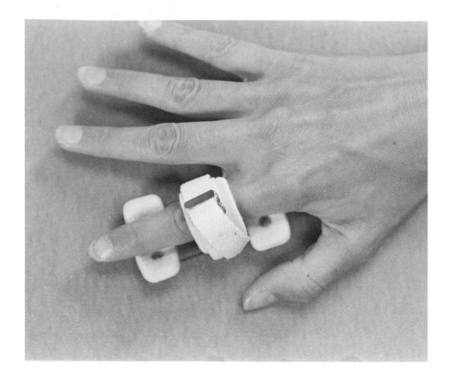

Type:	Dynamic, three-point pressure
Purpose:	To increase passive PIP joint extension (35° passively or less)

Indications:	Limited passive PIP extension following:
	    Soft-tissue injury
	    Arthrofibrosis secondary to trauma
	    PIP volar capsulectomy/capsulotomy
	    Flexor tenolysis

Wearing Times:	The safety pin splint is preferably worn as much as possible between exercises during the day and at night until the flexion contracture is resolved.
Precautions:	Watch for vascular compromise of the digit. Do not allow hyperextension of either the PIP or DIP joints. Watch for soft-tissue breakdown over the proximal phalanx. Not indicated when the dorsal aspect of the PIP joint is painful or the skin is of poor quality.

Correct Fit: Distal volar aspect of the splint is placed along the volar aspect of the DIP joint to prevent hyperextension of the distal phalanx. The proximal volar aspect of the splint is placed along the proximal base of the proximal phalanx.
The dorsal strap is placed slightly proximal to the PIP joint.
The tension is adjusted with the dorsal strap.

Available In: Sizes: small, medium, and large
These are prefabricated splints.

CAPENER SPLINT

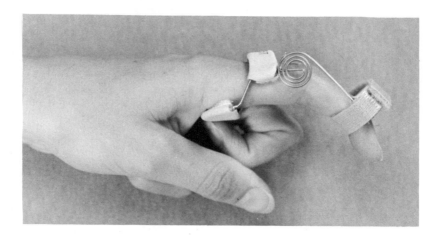

Type: Dynamic, three-point pressure

Purpose: To increase passive PIP joint extension (50° passively or less)
                      May assist a weak extensor mechanism at the PIP joint while
                      continuing to allow flexion of the digit

Indications: Limited active or passive PIP joint extension following:
                      Digital extensor tendon injury
                      Traumatic arthrofibrosis
                      Volar PIP joint capsulotomy/capsulectomy
                      Flexor tenolysis

Wearing Times: The Capener splint is preferably worn as much as possible be-
                      tween exercises during the day and at night until the flexion
                      contracture is resolved.

Precautions: Watch for discoloration or vascular compromise of the digit due
                      to a decrease in arterial or venous blood flow.
                      Do not allow hyperextension of either the PIP or DIP joints.
                      Watch for soft-tissue breakdown over the proximal phalanx.
                      Not indicated when the dorsal aspect of the PIP joint is painful
                      or the skin is irritated

Correct Fit: The proximal volar aspect is placed volarly under the base of
                      the proximal phalanx.
                      The middle bar lies dorsal and just proximal to the PIP joint.
                      The distal volar aspect should be secured proximal to the DIP
                      flexion crease.

Available In: Sizes: small, medium, large (long or short)
                      Large-short and medium-short are the sizes most commonly used
                      by the authors.
                      These are prefabricated splints.

JOINT JACK

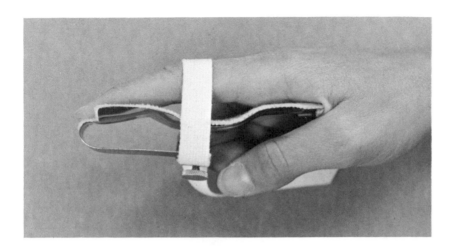

Type: Dynamic, three-point pressure

Purpose: To increase passive PIP joint extension with flexion contractures ≤35°.

Indications: Limited passive PIP extension following:
Soft-tissue injury
Traumatic arthrofibrosis

Wearing Times: The joint jack splint is preferably worn as much as possible between exercises during the day and at night.

Precautions: Do not allow hyperextension of either the PIP or DIP joints.

Correct Fit: The volar distal aspect supports the distal phalanx.
The volar proximal aspect supports the base of the proximal phalanx.
The dorsal strap is slightly proximal to the PIP joint.
Adjust the tension with the dorsal strap and volar screw.

Available In: Sizes: small and large
These are prefabricated splints.

SHORT DORSAL OUTRIGGER

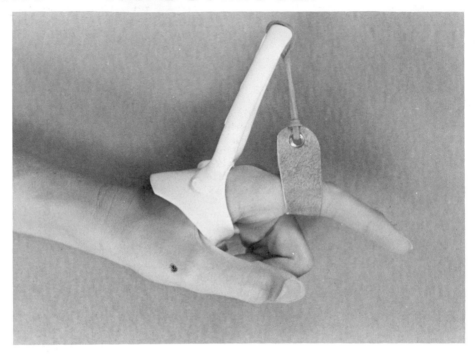

Type:	Dynamic, three-point pressure
Purpose:	To increase passive MP joint extension
Indications:	Arthrofibrosis secondary to crush or soft-tissue injury MP volar capsulectomy/capsulotomy MP arthroplasties in one or two digits (This splint is often worn with MP joint replacement arthroplasties following a traumatic injury.)
Wearing Times:	The splint is worn between exercises during the day. The splint may be worn at night or a static extension splint may be used. The splint is worn during exercise sessions and at all times of the day with MP arthroplasties
Precautions:	Potential pressure areas include the dorsum of the hand and along the first web space.
Correct Fit:	Rubber bands should be at a 90° angle from the outrigger to the proximal phalanx. Exception: MP arthroplasties for rheumatoid arthritis; see Chapter 6. The rubber bands' tension should be 8 ounces or less. (Note: With MP arthroplasties a minimal tension of 4 ounces should be applied.) The hypothenar portion of the splint must give adequate support to ensure stability of the outrigger. The palmar bar should connect in the palm.

SHORT DORSAL OUTRIGGER WITH LUMBRICAL BAR

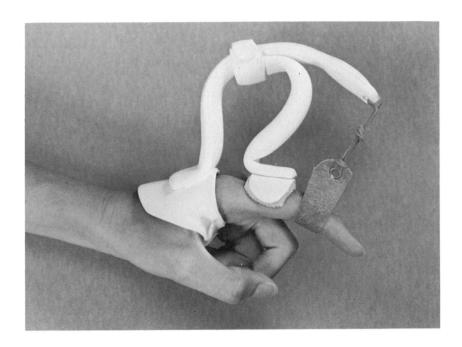

Type: Dynamic

Purpose: To increase passive PIP joint extension

Indications: PIP joint flexion contracture greater than 35° secondary to:
                   Arthrofibrosis of the PIP joint secondary to trauma
                   P_1 and P_2 fractures (once the fracture is clinically healed)
                   Subtotal palmar fasciectomy (if recurrence of the deformity
                   begins to develop)

Wearing Times: An average wearing time would be four times a day for 1-hour
                   sessions. The wearing times should be adjusted according to the
                   PIP joint extension deficit.
                   With chronic boutonnière deformities, once the PIP joint has
                   reached 0° passively, the PIP joint should be held at 0° for 8
                   weeks with a gutter splint or cylinder cast.

Precautions: Pressure points to be aware of include:
                   First web space
                   Dorsum of the proximal phalanx
                   Transverse palmar arch

Correct Fit: The lumbrical bar should have adequate length and stability to prevent MP hyperextension by holding the MP in 15° of flexion. The hypothenar portion of the splint must give adequate support to ensure stability of the outrigger.

The palmar bar should connect from the first web space to the hypothenar area.

Frequent adjustments (once or twice a week) are necessary to ensure correct line of pull.

The rubber bands should be at a 90° angle from the outrigger to the middle phalanx.

SPLINT FABRICATION FOR SHORT DORSAL OUTRIGGER WITH LUMBRICAL BAR

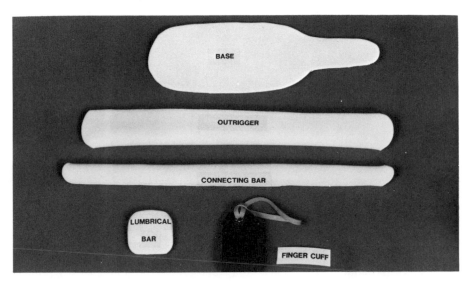

Components of the short dorsal outrigger with lumbrical bar. Suggested material—Orthoplast

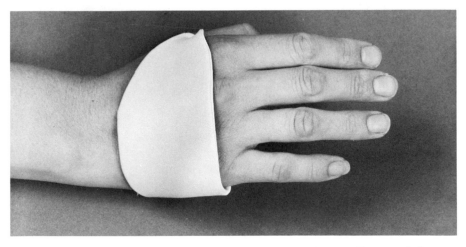

Step 1: The base is molded around the hand circumferentially. Watch for potential pressure in the first web space.

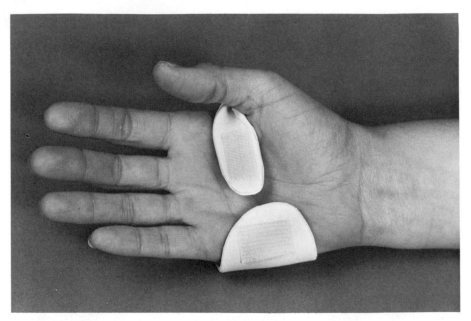

Step 2: The palmar piece should extend to the hypothenar area and connect to the palmar bar for maximum stability. It should be closed with 1-inch Velcro.

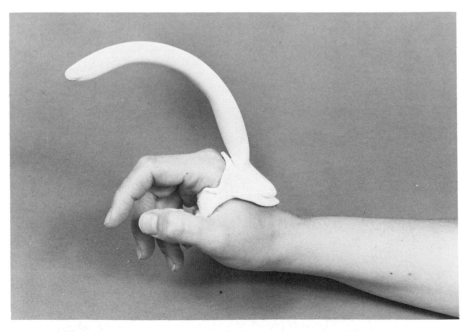

Step 3: The outrigger is adhered to the base. Placement of the outrigger is determined by the degree of joint contracture. A 90° line of pull from P_2 is essential.

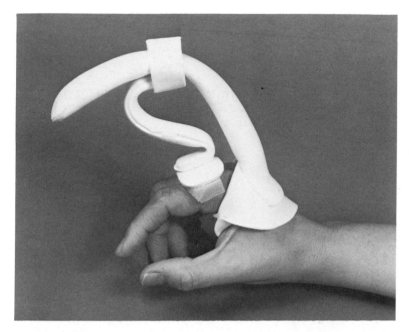

Step 4: The lumbrical bar is attached to the connector bar (which is tubed Orthoplast) by spot-heating it. The connector bar and the lumbrical bar prevent MP hyperextension, add strength to the outrigger, and direct the dynamic force to P_2.

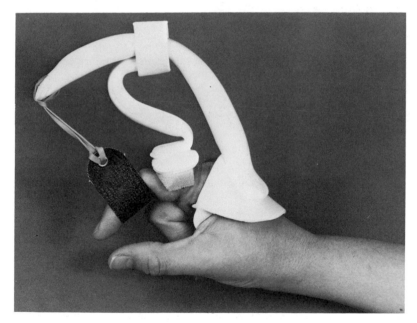

Step 5: A hole is punched through the outrigger with dynamic traction being extended from this point to the middle phalanx.

LONG DORSAL OUTRIGGER

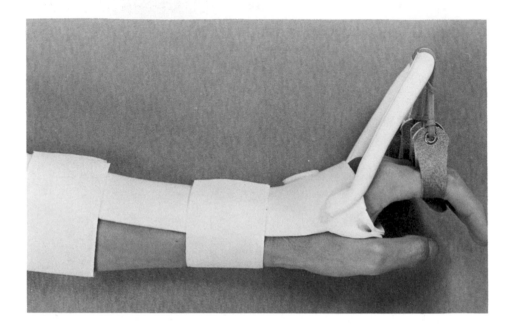

Type:	Dynamic with static wrist
Purpose:	To increase passive MP joint extension
Indications:	Limited passive extension of the MP joints following: Arthrofibrosis of the MP joints secondary to trauma Intrinsic contractures Metacarpal fractures (especially near the head and neck of the bone) Skin contractures of the palm secondary to skin grafting
Wearing Times:	The splint is generally worn four times a day for 1-hour sessions. The wearing times are adjusted according to the deficit.
Precautions:	Possible pressure points include: Dorsum of the hand Ulnar styloid First web space and the transverse palmar arch secondary to pressure from the palmar bar
Correct Fit:	The wrist is included to increase the stability of the splint by increasing the lever arm. The MP joints should not be allowed to hyperextend. The rubber bands should be at a 90° angle from the outrigger to the proximal phalanx.

LONG DORSAL OUTRIGGER WITH LUMBRICAL BAR

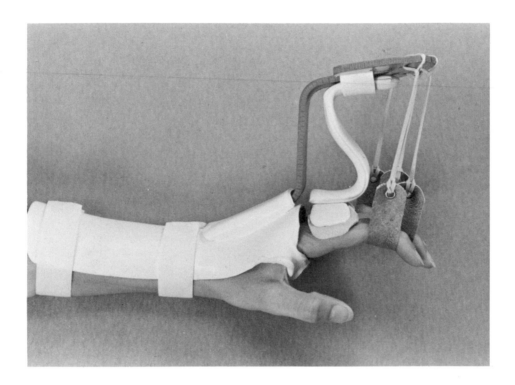

Type:	Dynamic with static wrist
Purpose:	To increase passive PIP extension To resolve extrinsic flexor tightness
Indications:	Limited passive extension of the PIP joints following: Arthrofibrosis of the PIP joints secondary to trauma Extrinsic flexor tightness Crush injuries with resultant PIP joint flexion contractures Median and/or ulnar nerve injury with resultant PIP joint flexion contractures
Wearing Times:	The splint is generally worn four times a day for 1-hour sessions. The wearing time is adjusted according to the flexion deformity.
Precautions:	Possible pressure points include: Dorsum of the hand The ulnar styloid Dorsum of the proximal phalanx Volar surface of the middle phalanx First web space

Correct Fit: The rubber bands should be at a 90° angle from the outrigger to the middle phalanx.

The lumbrical bar should have adequate length and stability to prevent hyperextension by maintaining the MP's in 15° of flexion.

Frequent adjustments (once or twice a week) are necessary to maintain the correct line of pull and maximize gains from the splinting program.

SPLINT FABRICATION FOR LONG DORSAL OUTRIGGER WITH LUMBRICAL BAR

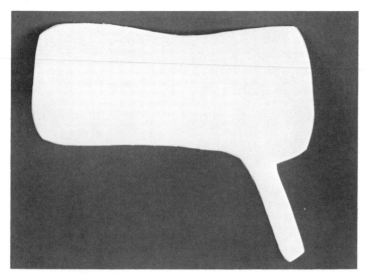

Step 1:   Design a dorsal wrist immobilization splint with palmar bar through the first web space. Suggested material: Orthoplast or Ultrasplint.

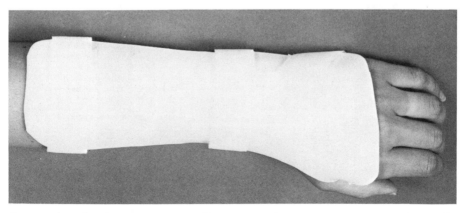

Step 2:   Fit the dorsal wrist immobilization splint to the patient's hand. Apply 1″ Velcro straps to secure the splint.

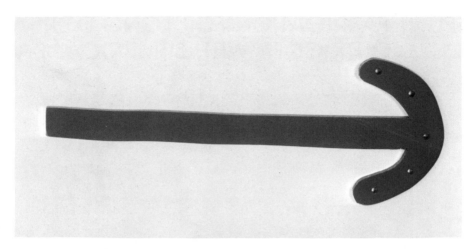

Step 3: Design the outrigger bar. The bar should contour in the same fashion as the middle phalanx of each digit does in relationship to one another. Suggested material: ⅜″ Kydex.

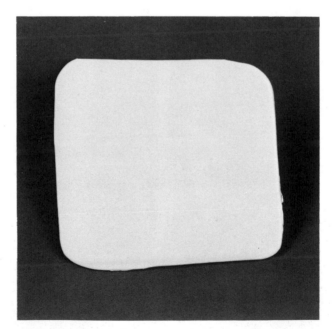

Step 4: Design the "pocket" for the outrigger (3″ × 4″) which will attach to the dorsal wrist immobilization splint. Suggested material: Orthoplast or Ultrasplint.

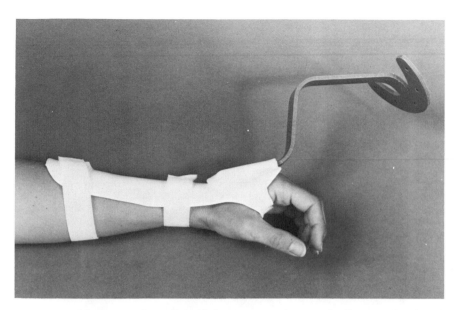

Step 5: Fold the "pocket" around the outrigger base and adhere to the dorsal wrist immobilization splint. The outrigger should then be spot-heated to the desired angle to allow for the 90° line of pull from P_2.

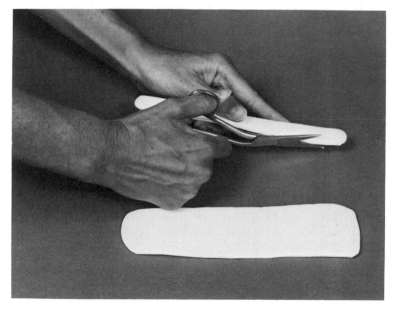

Step 6: To fabricate the connector bar use approximately a 2″ × 6″ piece of orthoplast and fold it back on itself. Then cut where the plastic meets to tube the material and seal it closed.

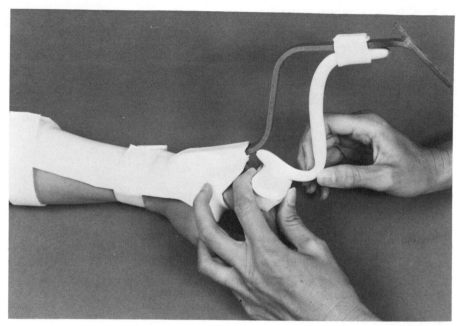

Step 7: Attach the connector bar to a lumbrical bar over P_1. The lumbrical bar is fabricated by contouring a doubly reinforced piece of Orthoplast along P_1 from the index to the small finger. The connector bar should be connected to the outrigger with orthoplast.

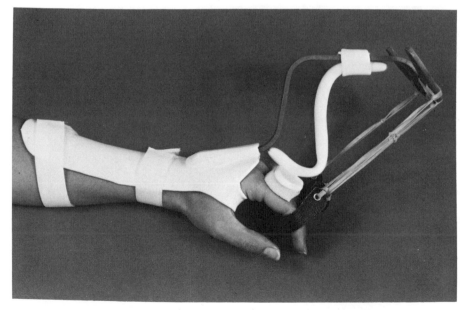

Step 8: For the dynamic traction, a 90° line of pull is necessary from the outrigger to the middle phalanx. #32 pure rubber bands are used with soft vinyl cuffs. Eight ounces of tension or less are recommended.

DIP MINIOUTRIGGER

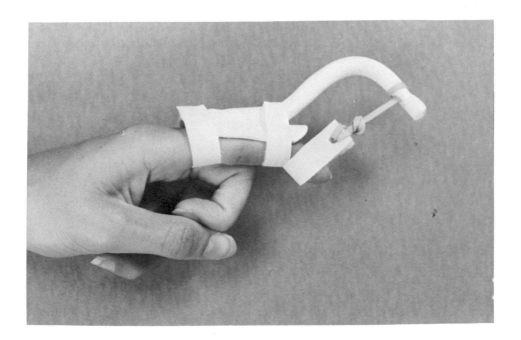

Type: Dynamic

Purpose: To increase passive DIP extension

Indications: Fixed flexion contracture of the DIP joint secondary to:
Chronic mallet deformity
Free tendon grafts
Arthrofibrosis secondary to trauma

Wearing Times: Ranges from 1-hour sessions, several times a day, to wearing the splint all the time between exercise sessions. This is determined by the extension deficit.
The splint should not be applied any earlier than 6 weeks after a free tendon graft.

Precautions: Watch for:
Distal slippage of the base of the splint
Pressure areas over the dorsum of the PIP joint and volar surface of the DIP joint.

Correct Fit: The PIP joint is held at neutral.
The dynamic force should be at a 90° angle from the outrigger to the distal phalanx.
Frequent adjustments (once or twice a week) are necessary to ensure the correct line of pull.

STATIC FINGER FLEXION SPLINTS 4

DORSAL BLOCKING SPLINT (DBS) TO PIP JOINT

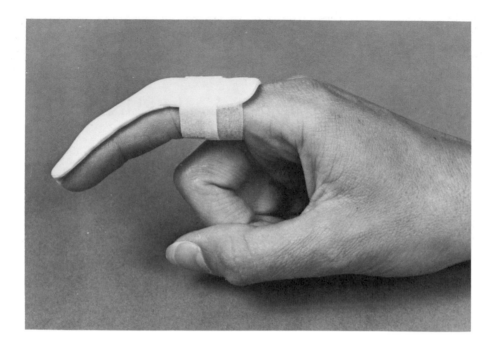

Type:	Static
Purpose:	To prevent full extension of the PIP joint yet allow for active and passive flexion exercises within the splint.
Indications:	Dorsal dislocations of the PIP joint (7 to 10 days post injury) (Note: ROM exercises are initiated between 7 and 10 days post-reduction.) The splint is worn continually for 6 weeks. Digital nerve repairs Volar plate avulsions Littler lateral band tenodesis
Wearing Times:	The splint is worn at all times for 6 weeks.
Precautions:	Watch for maceration over the dorsum of the PIP joint. Active extension of the PIP joint must not exceed the restraints of the splint.
Correct Fit:	The PIP joint is generally placed in 30° of flexion. The proximal strap must be secured just proximal to the PIP joint to prevent PIP extension beyond the restraints of the splint.

DORSAL EXTENSION BLOCK SPLINT: WRIST/MP/PIP/DIP JOINTS OF ALL DIGITS

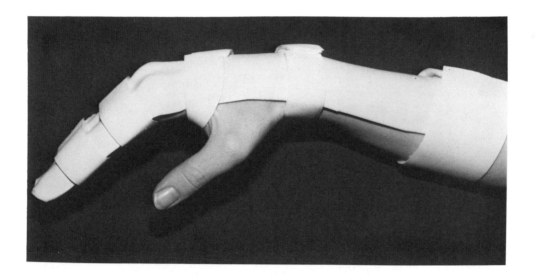

Type: Static

Purpose: Immobilization in a flexed posture to prevent tension on flexor tendon repair(s)

Indications: Flexor tendon repair(s) in zones 2 and 3
                   Forearm and hand flexor tendon repairs (frequently associated with median and/or ulnar nerve repair)

Wearing Times: The splint is worn continually for 5½ to 6 weeks following the repair.

Precautions: Possible pressure areas include:
                      Dorsum of the MP's and/or the PIP's
                      The ulnar styloid

Correct Fit: The wrist is placed in 20° of flexion with the MP's in 50° of flexion and the IP's in full extension.

SAFE-POSITION GUTTER

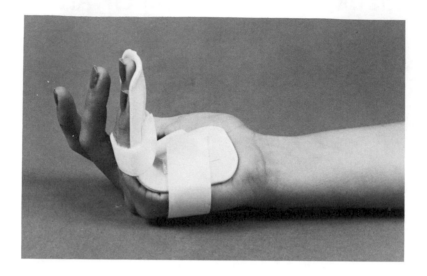

Type: Static

Purpose: This splint supports the digit in a "safe position" by placing the collateral ligaments on maximum stretch. This minimizes the probability of phalangeal joint contractures and stiffness.

Indications: Proximal phalanx fractures
Fractures of the metacarpal head, neck, or midshaft

Wearing Times: The splint is worn at all times until motion is initiated. Once ROM exercises are begun, the splint is worn between exercises and at night.

Correct Fit: The MP joints are held in 75° of flexion with the IP joints held in full extension.

DYNAMIC FINGER FLEXION SPLINTS 5

WRIST CUFF WITH MP SLINGS

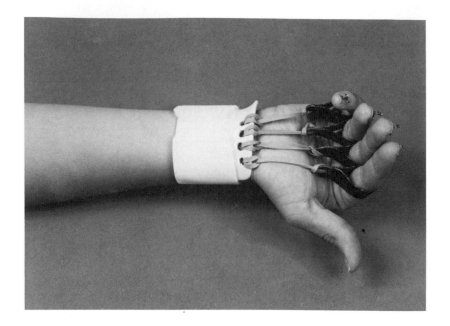

Type:	Dynamic
Purpose:	To increase or maintain passive MP flexion
Indications:	Limited passive MP flexion secondary to:
	Traumatic arthrofibrosis
	Phalangeal fractures (once clinically healed)
	Extensor tendon repair (a minimum of 6 weeks postoperatively)
	Extensor tenolysis and/or dorsal MP capsulotomies
Wearing Times:	The splint is generally worn four times a day for 1-hour sessions. The wearing times are adjusted by the passive limitation.
Precautions:	Watch for distal migration of the wrist cuff which may place pressure on the pisiform and/or the base of the first metacarpal.
Correct Fit:	The dynamic traction should be at a 90° angle to the proximal phalanx. The dynamic traction should be directed in the natural line of pull of the digits toward the scaphoid.

WRIST CUFF WITH IP CLIPS

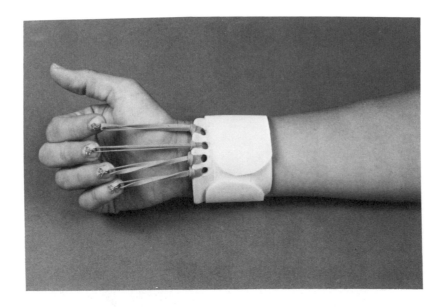

Type: Dynamic

Purpose: To increase or maintain passive MP and PIP flexion of the digits

Indications: Limited passive MP and PIP joint flexion secondary to:
Traumatic arthrofibrosis
Metacarpal and/or phalangeal fractures (once clinically healed)
Extensor tendon repairs (a minimum of 6 weeks postoperatively)
Extensor tenolysis and/or dorsal capsulectomy of the MP/PIP joints

Wearing Times: The splint is generally worn four times a day for 1-hour sessions with wearing times adjusted according to the passive flexion deficit.

Precautions: Watch for distal migration of the wrist cuff which may place pressure on the pisiform and/or base of the first metacarpal.

Correct Fit: The dynamic force should be directed in the natural line of pull of the digits toward the scaphoid.

WRIST CUFF WITH MP SLINGS AND IP CLIPS

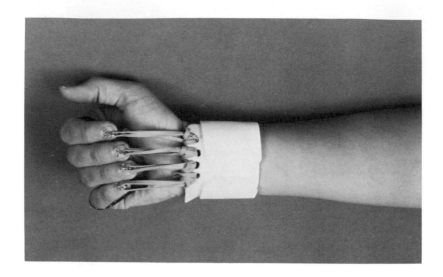

Type:	Dynamic
Purpose:	To increase passive MP and PIP motion of the digits with minimal passive assistance to the DIP joints
Indications:	Limited passive flexion of the digits secondary to: Traumatic arthrofibrosis Soft tissue crush injury Phalangeal fractures (once the fractures are clinically or radiographically healed) Extensor tendon repairs (a minimum of 6 weeks following repair) Dorsal MP, PIP capsulotomy, and/or extensor tenolysis of the hand
Wearing Time:	The splint is worn an average of three times a day for 45-minute sessions. If there is significant capsular or ligamentous tightness the splint should be worn for longer time frames.
Precautions:	Watch for: Circulatory problems and/or increased edema Excessive pressure along base of first metacarpal and/or pisiform Compression of the SBRN

Correct Fit: The base of the splint should rest just proximal to the distal wrist flexion crease.

The line of pull of the dynamic traction should be directed toward the scaphoid. This is the natural direction the digits follow with attempted flexion.

There should be comparable tension on the MP flexion cuffs and the IP clip.

Number 32 rubber bands are recommended for this splint.

The wrist cuff should have separate holes for each digit for the rubber band traction.

WRIST CUFF WITH PALMAR BAR

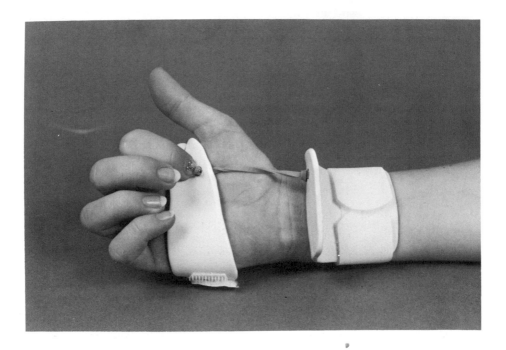

Type: Dynamic

Purpose: To increase passive PIP and DIP flexion with minimal passive
                         assistance to the MP joint

Indications: Limited passive flexion of the digits secondary to:
                            Arthrofibrosis of the MP, PIP, DIP joints secondary to trauma
                            Dorsal PIP, DIP capsulotomies
                            Phalangeal fractures (once clinically healed, an average of 6
                            weeks)
                            Digital extensor tenolyses
                            8 weeks after volar dislocation of the PIP joint

Wearing Time: This splint is usually worn three times a day for 30- to 45-minute
                         sessions.

Precautions: The considerations are the same as with a wrist cuff.

Correct Fit: The palmar bar should have separate holes for rubber band trac-
                         tion for each digit being mobilized.
                         Be sure the hole for the number 32 rubber band is large enough
                         to allow the rubber band to pull proximally in the hole.
                         The palmar bar must be designed so that motion is not blocked
                         at the MP joints. The splint should rest just proximal to the distal
                         palmar flexion crease to prevent this problem.

WRIST CUFF WITH MP BLOCK

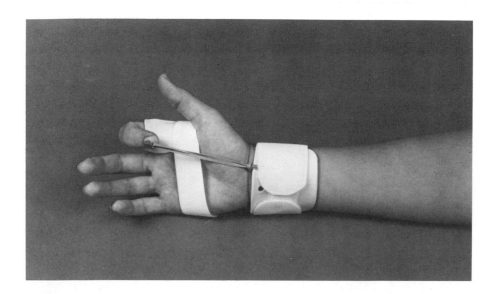

Type:	Dynamic with static MP block to prevent motion at the MP joint
Purpose:	To increase passive flexion of the PIP and/or DIP joints

Indications:	Limited passive IP joint motion secondary to:
	  Intrinsic tightness
	  Dorsal capsular or ligamentous tightness of the PIP/DIP joints

Contra-indications:	The splint is not indicated for extrinsic extensor tightness.
Precautions:	Watch for potential pressure areas along the volar surface of the PIP joint and the dorsum of the MP joint. The MP block may become too constricting if there is edema present. This may make removal of the MP block difficult.
Correct Fit:	The MP block should rest just proximal to the PIP joint and be contoured to prevent pressure in that area. The MP block should be "bubbled" over the dorsum of MP joint to prevent a potential pressure area. Dynamic traction should be directed in normal anatomical alignment toward the scaphoid.

WRIST IMMOBILIZATION
WITH MP SLINGS AND IP CLIPS

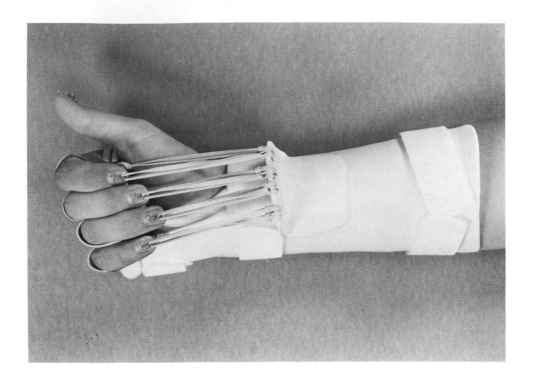

Type: Dynamic traction to the MP/PIP/DIP joints with static immobilization of the wrist

Purpose: To increase passive MP/PIP/DIP joint motion in a composite manner

Indications: Limited passive range of motion of the digits secondary to:
Extrinsic extensor tightness
(Note: The wrist may be placed in flexion up to 45° to aid in resolving the extrinsic extensor tightness.)
Arthrofibrosis of the MP, PIP, DIP joints secondary to hand trauma
Extensor tendon repairs (may be used 6 weeks after repair with careful observation for the development of an extensor lag)
Extensor tenolysis and/or dorsal MP, PIP, DIP capsulotomies
(Note: This splint may be indicated in place of a wrist cuff when the patient has a weak wrist and tends to flex the wrist palmarly while wearing the wrist cuff, when there is a need to place the wrist in a specific position, when the wrist must be protected and immobilized, or when a wrist cuff will not provide a 90° angle to the bone being mobilized.)

Precautions: Watch for distal slippage of the splint into the distal palmar flexion crease. The mechanics of the splint create this problem, which may be minimized by adding a strap to crisscross around a flexed elbow and attached to the proximal base of the splint. Do not place more than 8 ounces of tension on the rubber band traction and maintain equal tension on the MP slings and IP clips.

Correct Fit: The wrist immobilization portion of the splint should end just proximal to the distal palmar flexion crease.
A 90° line of pull is necessary from the bone being mobilized. The tension on the rubber bands should be 8 ounces or less.

SPLINT FABRICATION FOR WRIST IMMOBILIZATION SPLINT WITH MP SLINGS AND IP CLIPS

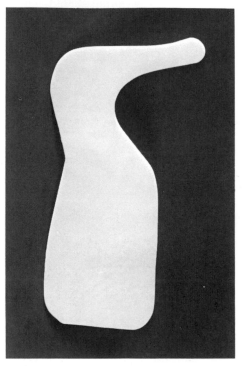

Step 1: Design a volar wrist immobilization splint with a bar which extends dorsally through the first web space. Suggested material: Polyform or Precision Splint.

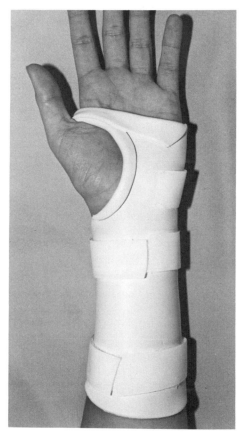

Step 2: Fabricate the volar wrist splint with the wrist at neutral or as indicated. Apply 1" Velcro straps to secure the splint.

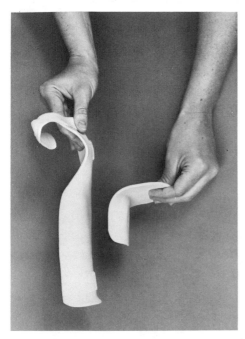

Step 3: Design the volar outrigger. It should be wide enough to accommodate the involved fingers and long enough to provide a 90° line of pull from P_1. It should be at least 3 inches long and be secured to the wrist immobilization splint.

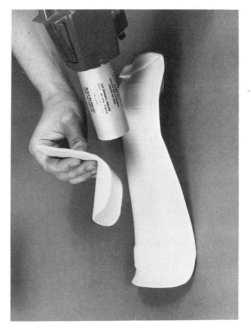

Step 4: Attach the outrigger to the volar wrist immobilization splint by heating both surfaces. Place the outrigger on the volar portion of the splint and mold the plastics together.

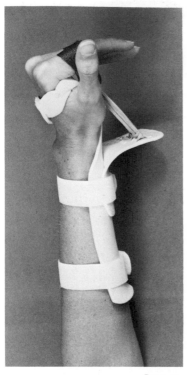

Step 5

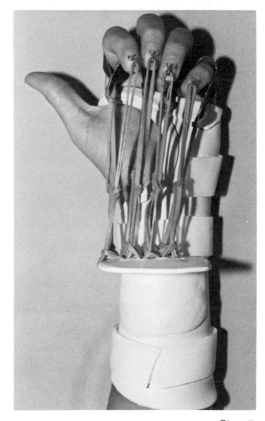

Step 6

Step 5: Attach the rubber bands with vinyl cuffs through punched holes in the outrigger. A 90° line of pull is necessary. Eight ounces of tension or less are recommended and there should be a slight radial pull directed toward the scaphoid.

Step 6: Glue small dress hooks onto the fingernails with Super Glue to allow for dynamic traction to the IP joints.

Step 7: Attach rubber bands to the outrigger through punched holes which provide a 90° line of pull. Eight ounces of tension or less should be applied with a slight radial pull towards the scaphoid.

Step 7

EXTRINSIC EXTENSOR SPLINT

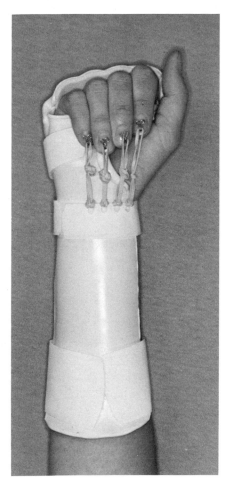 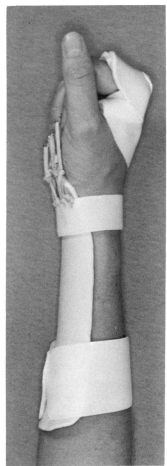

Type: Dynamic to the PIP and DIP joints with a static component to the wrist and MP joints

Purpose: To resolve extrinsic extensor tightness

Indication: Severe extrinsic tightness with significant rebound when performing passive flexion to the digits

Precautions: Be sure to not place pressure along the SBRN at the wrist.
Watch for distal slippage of the splint. It may be necessary to add a strap around the elbow to minimize this problem.
Watch for pressure areas along the dorsum of each proximal phalanx.

Wearing Time: The problem of extrinsic extensor tightness is usually paramount when it occurs. For this reason, wearing the splint at all times between exercise sessions is not uncommon.

Correct Fit: Be sure to leave ample space proximal to the distal palmar flexion crease to prevent blocking MP motion of the digits.
The wrist is placed in the appropriate amount of flexion which is determined by the amount of extrinsic tightness.
The dorsal P_1 block is well-contoured over the entire surface of each proximal phalanx.
The appropriate amount of tension (≤ 8 ounces) is placed on the rubber band traction and at a 90° angle to the bone being mobilized. The outrigger is fitted just proximal to the wrist strap to allow for a correct line of pull.
A disadvantage of this splint is that it requires significant adjustments with each return visit due to the progress made in resolving the extrinsic extensor tightness.

DUKE VELCRO

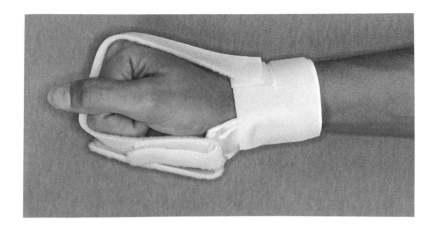

Type: Static with dynamic adjustment to increase passive flexion of the digits

Purpose: To increase passive MP and PIP motion of the digits

Indications: Limited passive flexion of the IP's where there is:
  Absence of the fingernail such as with DIP amputations
  Loss of fingernail integrity following a crush injury
  A hypersensitive nail that makes dynamic traction with a fingernail clip intolerable
Patients with poor vascular supply to the digits (e.g., those with diabetes, digital replants)

Precautions: Watch for distal slippage of the wrist strap.
The wrist strap may cause edema due to its circumferential nature.

Wearing Times: The splint is worn, on the average, three to four times a day for 30-minute sessions.

Correct Fit: The wrist cuff should stay proximal to the distal wrist flexion crease.
The dorsal straps should originate from the dorsum of the wrist strap and be brought distally over the MP and PIP joints and secured to the volar side of the wrist strap.
Over the midportion of the proximal phalanx, a loose circumferential strap should be fitted to keep the strap in proper alignment and prevent slippage laterally.
Individual straps should be applied to each digit and the line of pull directed toward the scaphoid.

COMBINATION SPLINTS 6

SINGLE WYNN-PARRY

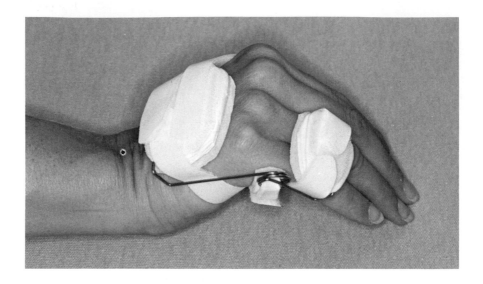

Type: Dynamic

Purpose: This splint prevents MP hyperextension of the ring and small fingers which secondarily allows for full IP extension by mechanically correcting the claw deformity. If the splint is worn continuously for approximately 1 year the volar plates will tighten and often prevent the need for tendon transfers to correct the claw deformity.

Indication: Ulnar nerve palsy

Precautions: The patient should avoid machinery in which the coils could get caught.

Wearing Times: The splint should be worn continuously, 24 hours a day, for approximately 1 year, but be removed for bathing.

Correct Fit: MP hyperextension must be prevented by the splint.
The resting posture of the hand in the splint is 45° of MP flexion.
The coil should be aligned with the small finger MP joint which is the axis of rotation for the joint.
The palmar bar should be well-molded to the transverse arch of the hand, along the distal palmar flexion crease.

SPLINT FABRICATION FOR SINGLE WYNN-PARRY

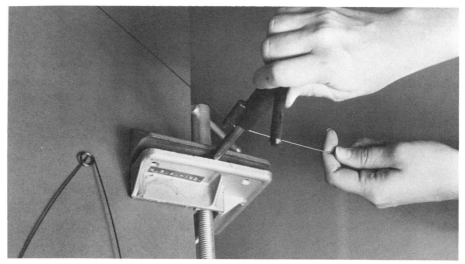

Step 1: Using a 14″ piece of 22-gauge piano wire, coil it in the center (two full turns) with a wire jig.

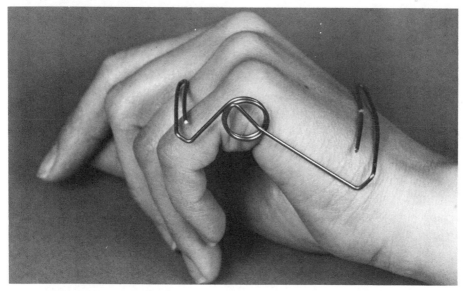

Step 2: Align coil at axis of MP joint and shape wire proximally and distally over the dorsum of the hand, contouring to the hand arches. The distal portion should fall at P_1 of the affected digits and the proximal wire should lay transversely over the midmetacarpal level, spanning the width of the hand to the third metacarpal.

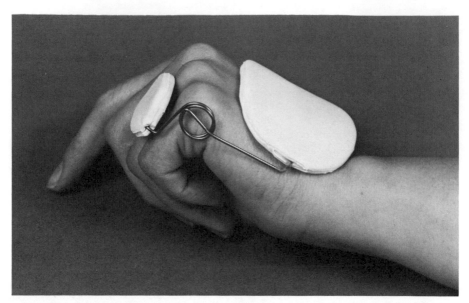

Step 3: Apply splinting material, double-thickness, over the wires on the dorsum of the metacarpals and P_1 of the involved digits. The proximal portion should be large enough to provide stability.

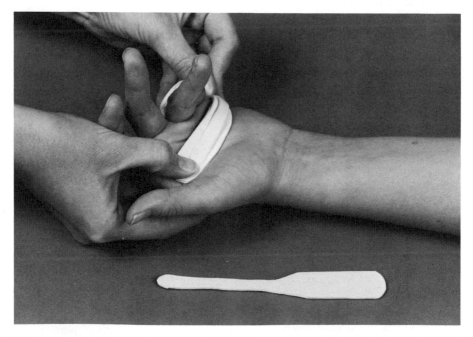

Step 4: A long narrow piece of splint material is passed through the coil, doubled back onto itself, and formed to the transverse metacarpal arch. Be sure to keep the coil in line with the axis of the MP joint.

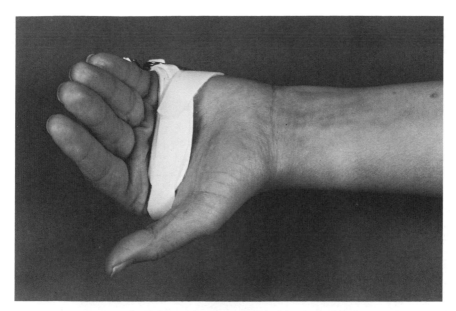

Step 5: A strap is attached from the palmar bar, through the first web space, and attached to the proximal dorsal portion of the splint.

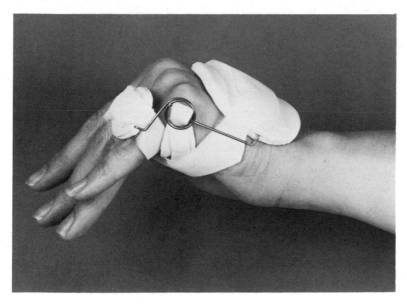

Step 6: Another strap is attached at the distal portion of the splint, wrapped around the involved digits at P_1, and then attached to the splint to stabilize the distal portion of the splint during motion.

DOUBLE WYNN-PARRY

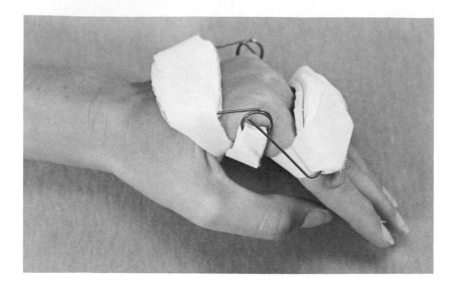

Type: Dynamic

Purpose: This splint prevents MP hyperextension of the index, long, ring, and small fingers which secondarily facilitates active IP extension of each digit. This prevents the claw deformity posture which results from the combined median and ulnar nerve palsy.

Indications: Combined median and ulnar nerve palsy in which clawing is apparent and the joints are passively supple

Precautions: The splint should not be worn near machinery in which it might get caught.

Wearing Times: The splint must be worn continuously, 24 hours a day, for up to 1 year to be effective in tightening the volar plates.

Correct Fit: MP hyperextension must be prevented by the splint.
The resting posture of the hand in the splint is 45° of MP flexion.
The coil should be aligned with the small finger MP joint that is the axis of rotation for the joint.
The palmar bar should be well-molded to the transverse arch of the hand, along the distal palmar flexion crease.

RHEUMATOID ARTHRITIS (RA) SPLINT: POSTOPERATIVE SPLINT FOR MP JOINT REPLACEMENT ARTHROPLASTIES

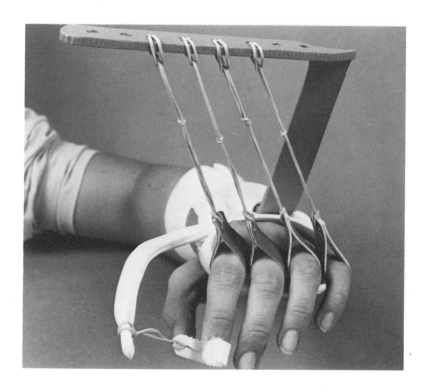

Type: Dynamic

Purpose: This splint positions the MP joints in normal anatomical alignment (neutral alignment) following MP arthroplasties for rheumatoid arthritis. The rubber band traction assists with MP extension and radial deviation and allows for controlled flexion of the digits.

The "supinator" is included to prevent pronation of the index finger. This may occur secondary to having the collateral ligament of the index MP joint reconstructed at the time of the MP arthroplasties.

Indications: MP arthroplasties or synovectomies for rheumatoid arthritis

Precautions: Do not allow the MP's to hyperextend (be especially watchful of the small finger MP).

Watch for skin irritation and pressure areas. This problem is easily created because of the rheumatoid patient's fragile skin.

71

Wearing Time: The splint should be applied 3 to 5 days after surgery over a light compressive dressing. The splint is worn continuously throughout the day. A resting pan splint is fabricated for night wear. The RA splint is worn for 10 to 12 weeks following surgery.

Correct Fit: The MP slings should be directed radially from the outrigger to the proximal phalanx at approximately a 60° angle. The desired positioning is neutral alignment of the metacarpophalangeal joints.

The palmar bar must support the transverse metacarpal arch and travel across the palm to the fifth metacarpal.

Approximately 4 ounces of tension is ideal for the rubber band traction from the outrigger. Even less tension is required for the small finger since it has the greatest tendency to hyperextend.

The "supinator" should be positioned on the radial border of the distal aspect of the RA splint, approximately 3 inches from the distal phalanx. The Velcro tab is directed volar to the fingertip and attached on the nail.

WRIST IMMOBILIZATION WITH MP SLINGS AND IP EXTENSION GUTTERS

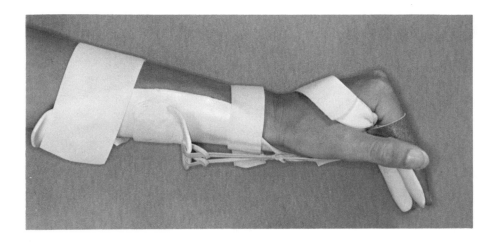

Type: Static to the wrist, PIP, and DIP joints
Dynamic to the MP joints

Purpose: The splint dynamically positions the digits in the safe or intrinsic plus position. This position maintains the collateral ligaments on maximum stretch which minimizes or prevents joint contractures.

Indications: Extensor tenolysis over the dorsum of the hand and digit(s), often combined with dorsal MP and PIP capsulotomies
Soft-tissue crush injuries
Crush injuries with phalangeal fractures

Precautions: Watch for distal slippage of the wrist-immobilizing portion of the splint.
When edema is present, use the widest straps possible to minimize the swelling.
When the splint is fitted during the first week of a crush injury, the edema must be monitored closely.
Tension may need to be reduced on the rubber band traction if pain and edema are significant.

Wearing Times: The splint is generally worn between exercise sessions and at night.

Correct Fit: A 90° line of pull is necessary to the proximal phalanx.
8 ounces of tension or less should be used on the rubber band traction.
The gutters may be held secure with paper tape instead of Velcro straps.
The wrist is placed in 25° dorsiflexion, the MP joints in maximum flexion, and the IP joints in full extension.

WRIST IMMOBILIZATION SPLINT WITH MP FLEXION BLOCK

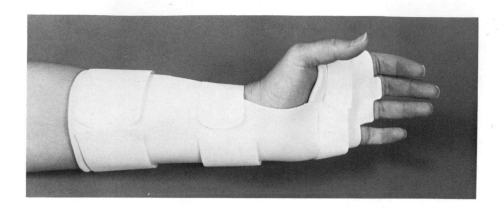

Type: Static

Purpose: To prevent wrist and MP joint motion
To allow active and passive PIP and DIP flexion

Indications: Extensor tendon repairs proximal to the MP joint level
Intrinsic tightness
Intrinsic releases (postoperatively)
The splint may be used for exercise to isolate the FDS and FDP.
(Note: This splint has been especially helpful following forearm and digital flexor tenolyses in which the patient is generating poor excursion of the long flexors and is primarily flexing at the level of the MP joint.)

Wearing Times: With intrinsic releases, the splint is worn at all times between exercise sessions for 8 weeks.
With extensor tendon repairs, the splint is worn continuously for 4½ weeks before range-of-motion exercise sessions are initiated.

Correct Fit: The wrist and MP's are held in neutral alignment for the indications listed above.
The distal end of the splint must rest just proximal to the PIP joints.
(Note: The wrist and MP's are held in full extension whenever the splint's purpose is to exercise and isolate the long flexors.)

RESTING PAN

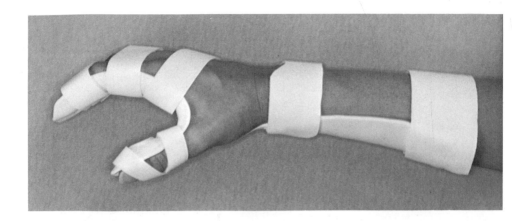

Type: Static

Purpose: To immobilize the wrist, digits, and thumb in a functional position

Indications: Crush injuries in which there have been simultaneous flexor and extensor tendon repairs
Edema and inflammatory problems of the hand of unknown or questionable cause
Infections of the hand
Replants of the hand/digits

Precautions: Due to the static nature of the splint, be sure the patient exercises at frequent intervals once ROM exercises are initiated.

Wearing Times: With crush injuries, the splint is generally initiated at 3½ weeks or when active ROM of the digit is allowed.
With edema, inflammatory conditions, and infections, the splint is worn until the symptoms begin to subside.
(Note: once the symptoms begin to resolve, the splint should be removed a minimum of 3 times a day for active and passive ROM exercises.)

Correct Fit: Wide straps should be applied in all cases.
The wrist is positioned in 25° of dorsiflexion, the MP's in 45° flexion, and the PIP and DIP joints in 25° of flexion. The thumb should be in 45° of abduction and slightly flexed.

SAFE POSITION SPLINT, WRIST INCLUDED

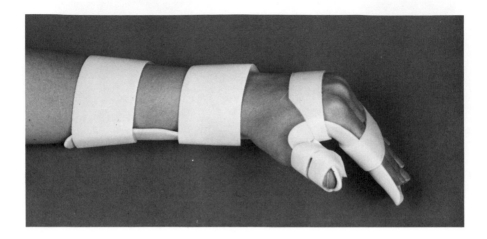

Type: Static

Purpose: This splint is used to prevent MP joint extension contractures and PIP joint flexion contractures often seen secondary to crush injuries and phalangeal fractures.

Indications:
Metacarpal fractures
Proximal phalanx fractures
Soft-tissue crush injuries
Second- and third-degree burns
Dorsal MP capsulotomies

Wearing Time: The splint is worn between exercises and at night. Exercise times are determined based on healing of the injured area.

Precautions: The straps should have a wide area of application to minimize the edema.

Correct Fit: The MP joints are placed in maximum flexion with the IP joints in full extension. This places the collateral ligaments of these joints on maximum stretch.
The splint should hold the wrist in 25° of dorsiflexion, the MP's at approximately 75° of flexion, and the IP's in full extension. The thumb is placed midway between radial and palmar abduction.

THUMB SPLINTS 7

WEB SPACER

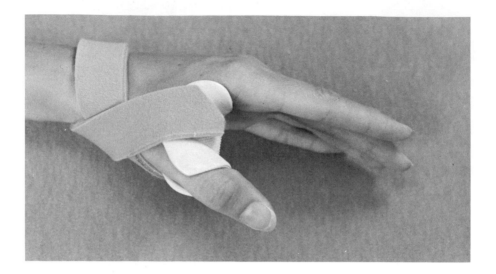

Type:	Static
Purpose:	This splint is used to maintain the first web space. It may also be used to increase serially the passive abduction of the thumb and/or increase extension of the thumb MP joint.

Indications:	The splint prevents or attempts to correct first web space contractures resulting from:
	    Crush injuries
	    Burns
	    Disuse
	    Myostatic contracture of the thumb intrinsics
	    Median nerve injury (motor component)
	The splint is often used 6 weeks after a trapezial arthroplasty for protection and when there is a slight contracture of the web space.

Wearing Time:	When using serially, the splint is often worn between exercises and at night. It must be adjusted or changed weekly until the abduction/extension matches the uninvolved thumb, or progress plateaus. With acute low median nerve palsies, the web spacer is generally worn only at night.
Precautions:	When one is serially increasing abduction, the force should be directed to the CMC joint and care should be taken that the MP joint ulnar collateral ligament is not significantly stretched.
Correct Fit:	The web spacer should be fitted so that it does not extend beyond the distal palmar flexion crease, which would block index MP flexion. Generally, the splint only immobilizes the thumb MP joint unless the EPL or the IP joint requires protection.

DYNAMIC THUMB FLEXION SPLINT WITH CMC IMMOBILIZATION

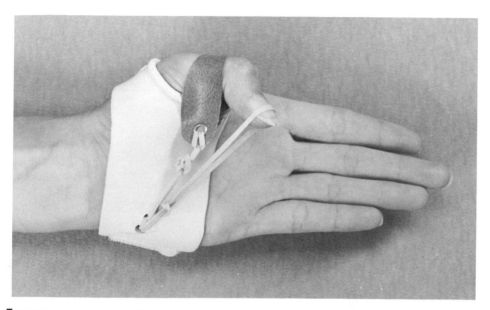

Type: Dynamic

Purpose: This splint may be used to:
Increase passive MP and IP joint motion by mobilizing the tight dorsal capsules of these joints
Mobilize extension contractures of the MP and IP joints of the thumb
Immobilize and protect the CMC joint as the dynamic traction is applied to the MP and IP joints

Indications: Arthrofibrosis of the MP and IP joints of the thumb
Soft-tissue injuries of the thumb
Clinically healed fractures of the thumb
EPL repairs (a minimum of 6 weeks postoperatively)
MP and IP dorsal capsulotomies of the thumb
Trapezial arthroplasties (7 weeks postoperatively)

Wearing Time: The wearing time is contingent upon the severity of arthrofibrosis or capsular stiffness. On an average, the splint is worn four times a day for 30- to 45-minute sessions.

Precautions: Care should be taken that the CMC joint is properly immobilized to prevent excessive rotary forces. The effectiveness of the splint is diminished if this is not accomplished.

Correct Fit: The thumb should be brought into composite flexion with the CMC being adequately immobilized.
MP flexion should not be restricted by the splint.
A 90° line of pull from the phalanx being mobilized is necessary.

SPLINT FABRICATION FOR DYNAMIC THUMB FLEXION SPLINT WITH CMC IMMOBILIZATION

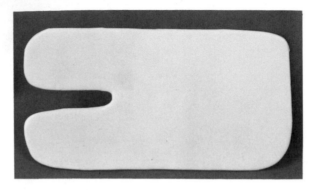

Step 1: Cut out a modified "U"-shaped pattern. (Suggested material: Polyform or Precision Splint)

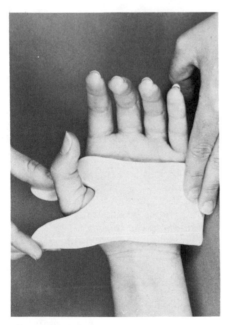

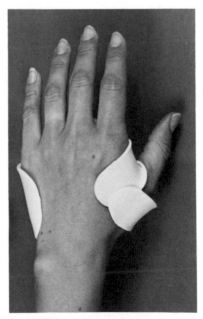

Step 2: Fit the splint volarly with the base of the "U" wrapping around the thenar eminence of the thumb just below the MP flexion crease. Flare all edges along the thumb and distal palmar flexion crease.

Step 3: Continue wrapping the distal edges of the "U" around to the dorsum of the hand until they meet. The hypothenar edge is wrapped around dorsally for support as well.

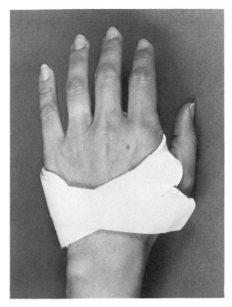

Step 4: Velcro straps are applied in a criss-cross fashion on the dorsum of the hand.

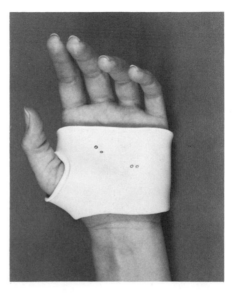

Step 5: For dynamic traction, a 90° line of pull is necessary from the proximal and distal phalanges of the thumb to the splint. Line up the rubber band traction from the proximal and distal phalanx and mark the splint.

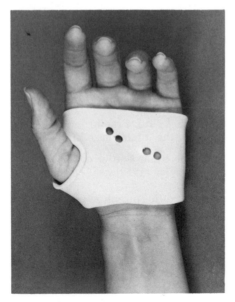

Step 6: Using a leather hole punch, double holes are placed as marked on the splint.

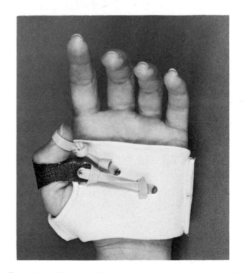

Step 7: Dynamic traction is applied using #73 pure rubber bands with a leather cuff attached for the MP joint. Approximately 8 ounces of tension or less should be applied.

WRIST CUFF WITH MP SLING AND IP CLIP

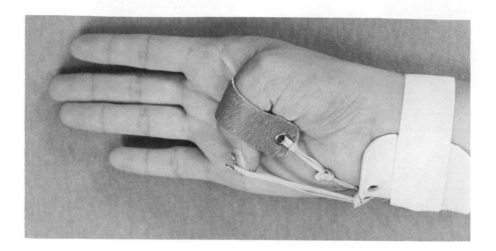

Type: Dynamic

Purpose: This splint is used to increase passive flexion to the thumb MP and IP joints as well as the CMC joint.

Indications: Arthrofibrosis
Soft-tissue trauma
Clinically healed fractures of the thumb
EPL repair (a minimum of 6 weeks postoperatively)
MP and/or IP dorsal capsulotomies

Wearing Time: The amount of wearing time should be determined by the severity of arthrofibrosis, tendon tightness, or capsular stiffness. An average wearing schedule would be three times a day for 45-minute sessions.

Precautions: Watch for distal slippage of the splint. Pressure may occur on the pisiform and potentially on the ulnar nerve in this area.

Correct Fit: The wrist cuff is placed on the ulnar border of the wrist and formed to the midline of the volar and dorsal surfaces of the wrist.
A 90° line of pull is necessary to the proximal and distal phalanges.

SHORT OPPONENS

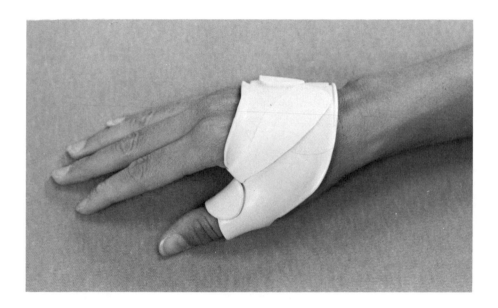

Type: Static

Purpose: This splint is used to position and immobilize the thumb MP
                     joint while allowing thumb IP motion. The thumb is positioned
                     in palmar abduction.

Indications: Radial collateral ligament strain of the thumb MP joint
                     Ulnar collateral ligament strain of the thumb MP joint
                     Median nerve injury: to hold the thumb in functional position
                     MP joint dorsal dislocations (7 to 10 days post injury)
                     Nondisplaced metacarpal or proximal phalanx fractures of the
                     thumb where minimal support/protection is required

Wearing Time: With acute injuries, the splint is generally worn continuously
                     for 3 weeks.
                     When the motor component of the median nerve is interrupted,
                     the splint is worn to enhance hand function and maintain the
                     first web space.

Precautions: The splint should not place excessive strain on the UCL. This
                     is accomplished by placing the thumb in 45° of palmar abduction
                     or less.

Correct Fit: The ulnar side of the splint should wrap around and extend to
                     the fourth metacarpal. If the splint is to be worn for dislocation
                     of the MP joint, the MP joint should be placed in 30° of flexion.

WRIST AND THUMB STATIC (IP FREE) (THUMB SPICA SPLINT)

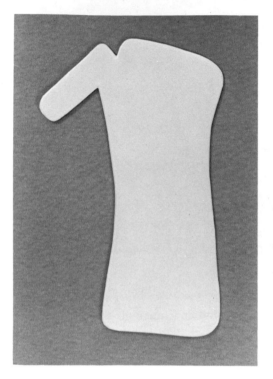 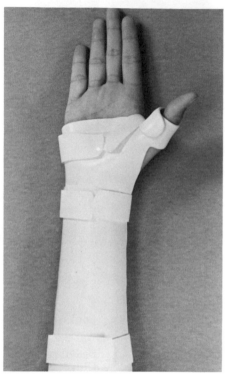

Type:	Static
Purpose:	This splint is used to immobilize the wrist, CMC, and MP joints of the thumb.
Indications:	DeQuervain's tenosynovitis Trapezial replacement arthroplasties Painful basilar joint arthritis Radial or ulnar collateral ligament strain or reconstruction of the MP joint
Wearing Time:	In conservative treatment of DeQuervain's tenosynovitis and basilar joint arthritis, the splint is worn continuously for 3 to 4 weeks. At that time the patient is reevaluated to determine if the pain is resolving. For RCL/UCL reconstruction, the splint is worn continuously for 6 weeks.

Precautions: The splint should not hold the thumb in palmar abduction greater than 45°, which would create excessive stress on the UCL of the MP joint. Be sure the radial side of the splint does not compress the SBRN.

Correct Fit: The wrist should be placed in 15° dorsiflexion, the thumb in approximately 45° of abduction, and the thumb MP joint in 15° of flexion.

Care should be taken that the splint ends at the distal palmar flexion crease, thus allowing full digital flexion. In addition, the thumb piece wrapped circumferentially around the proximal phalanx of the thumb should allow full IP joint motion. This portion of the splint should be secured with Velcro to allow for fluctuation in edema and easy removal of the splint.

WRIST AND THUMB STATIC (IP INCLUDED)

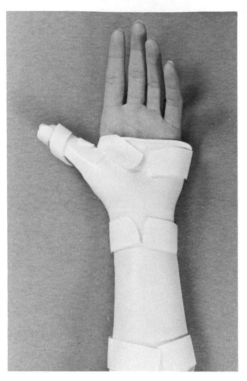 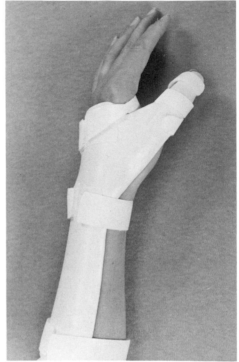

Type: Static

Purpose: This splint is used to immobilize the wrist and thumb either in a dorsal or volar fashion.

Indications: The dorsal application is used postoperatively for:
                 Opponensplasty
                 FPL repair
                 Adductorplasty
                 Tendon transfers for FPL function
                 The volar application is used for:
                 EPL repair
                 Tendon transfers for EPL function
                 Extrinsic flexor tightness of the thumb
                 Extensor tenolysis of the thumb
                 Flexor tenolysis of the thumb

Wearing Time: Dorsal application
                 For opponensplasties, adductorplasties, delayed mobilization of FPL repairs, and FPL tendon transfers, the splint is worn continuously from the 3rd to the 6th week postoperatively; both active and passive range-of-motion exercises are initiated

within the splint at 3 weeks. The splint is discontinued at 6 weeks.

Volar application

For extensor transfers to the thumb and EPL repairs, the splint is fitted 4 weeks postoperatively and worn between ROM exercises and at night. The splint is discontinued at 6 weeks providing full extension is present.

For flexor tightness of the FPL, the splint is worn between exercises and at night until the flexor tightness is resolved.

Following extensor or flexor tenolysis the splint is worn between exercises and at night for approximately 6 weeks.

Precautions: Care should be taken to avoid potential pressure points such as the:

Ulnar styloid
Superficial branch of the radial nerve
Thumb MP joint (dorsal application)
MP joints of the digits (dorsal application)

Correct Fit: Dorsal application

For opponensplasties, FPL repairs, and tendon transfers for flexion of the thumb, the wrist should be held in 30° of flexion and the thumb positioned in palmar abduction and slight flexion. For adductorplasties, the wrist is held at neutral and the thumb is placed in 30° abduction.

Volar application

For EPL repairs, tendon transfers for thumb extension, and extensor tenolysis of the thumb, the wrist is placed in 15° to 20° of dorsiflexion with the thumb in full extension.

For extrinsic flexor tightness of the thumb the wrist and thumb are placed in full extension.

WRIST SPLINTS 8

WRIST IMMOBILIZATION SPLINT

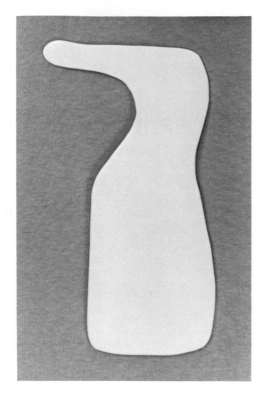 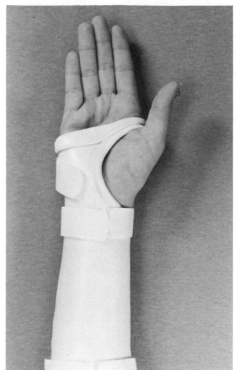

Type: Static

Purpose: This splint is used to immobilize the wrist for protection, comfort, or to quiet inflammation.

Indications: Carpal tunnel syndrome (0 to 15° dorsiflexion)
FCU/FCR tendonitis (0 to 15° palmar flexion)
Total wrist arthroplasty (At three weeks postoperatively it is fitted to wear between exercise sessions.)
Radial nerve palsy (30° dorsiflexion)
Volar or dorsal wrist ganglion (0 to 15° dorsiflexion)
Colles' fracture (When the cast is removed, it is worn between exercise sessions.)
Nondisplaced metacarpal fractures (proximal base)

Wearing Time: For acute injuries, inflammation, or carpal tunnel syndrome, the splint is worn continuously until the symptoms subside or surgery is indicated.

Precautions: Areas that must be monitored include:
Distal migration of the splint
Compression of the superficial branch of the radial nerve
Pressure points such as the:
   Ulnar styloid
   Volar and dorsal aspect of the index MP joint
   First web space
   Dorsum of the metacarpals

Correct Fit: The splint should hold the wrist securely yet allow full finger and thumb motion.

TENNIS ELBOW SPLINT

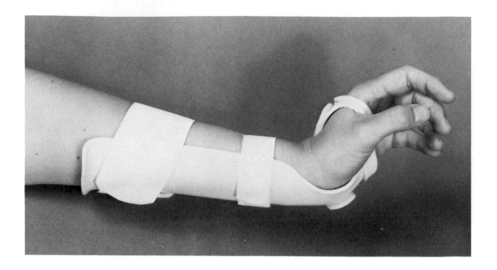

Type: Static

Purpose: To immobilize the wrist in 45° of dorsiflexion which minimizes stress to the extensor carpi radialis brevis

Indications: Lateral epicondylitis, "tennis elbow" (may also present with radial tunnel syndrome)

Wearing Time: The splint is worn continuously for 3 to 6 weeks. The patient is then re-evaluated to determine the effectiveness of the splint in resolving the symptoms. This is determined by the physician.

Precautions: Areas which should be monitored include:
Distal migration of the splint
Compression of the superficial branch of the radial nerve
Pressure points such as the:
     Ulnar styloid
     Volar and dorsal aspect of index MP joint
     First web space
     Dorsum of the metacarpals

Correct Fit: The splint should hold the wrist securely in 45° of dorsiflexion. The digits and thumb should be free for full range of motion.

DORSAL WRIST EXTENSION BLOCK SPLINT

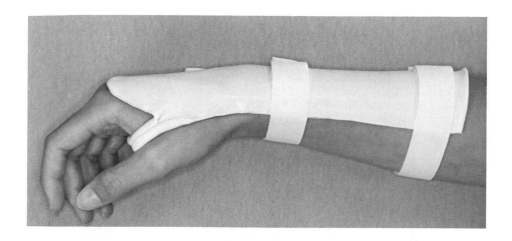

Type: Static

Purpose: The splint is worn to prevent extension of the wrist and yet allow
active flexion and extension of the digits.

Indications: The splint is worn with median and ulnar nerve repairs and/or
repairs of the wrist flexors (FCU, FCR, PL).

Wearing Time: The splint is worn continuously for 6 weeks from the date of the
repair.

Precautions: Potential areas for pressure points include:
Ulnar styloid
Dorsum of the MP joints
First web space
Transverse palmar arch

Correct Fit: For wrist flexor tendon repairs combined with nerve repairs, the
splint should initially hold the wrist securely in 30° of palmar
flexion. Wrist extension should be increased by 10° increments
from the 3rd to the 6th week.

DYNAMIC WRIST EXTENSION SPLINT

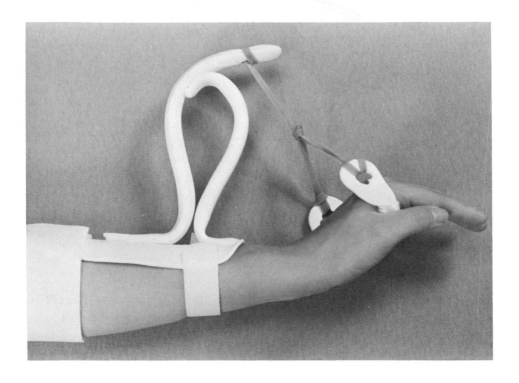

Type: Dynamic

Purpose: This splint is worn to increase passive wrist extension.

Indications: Colles' fracture (once the fracture is clinically healed)
Total wrist arthroplasty (a minimum of 6 weeks postoperatively)
Arthrofibrosis of the wrist

Wearing Time: The splint is worn an average of four times a day for 1-hour sessions; wearing time is adjusted according to the deficit.

Precautions: Potential pressure points include:
  Ulnar styloid
  First web space

Correct Fit: The traction force should be at a 90° line of pull from the meta-carpals with the rotary force at the distal carpal row.
Care should be taken that the outrigger is centrally located so that the wrist is extended in a midline axis.
The distal base of the splint should not block wrist dorsiflexion.

DYNAMIC WRIST FLEXION SPLINT

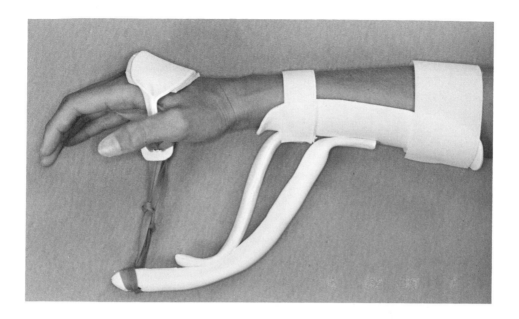

Type: Dynamic

Purpose: This splint is worn to increase passive wrist flexion.

Indications: Colles' fracture (once the fracture is clinically healed)
Total wrist arthroplasty (a minimum of 6 weeks postopera-
tively)
Ganglionectomy (dorsal)
Arthrofibrosis following soft-tissue trauma

Wearing Time: The splint is worn an average of four times a day for 1-hour
sessions; wearing time is adjusted according to the deficit.

Precautions: Potential pressure areas include:
First web space
Superficial branch of the radial nerve
Dorsum of the hand

Correct Fit: The traction force should be at a 90° line of pull from the metacarpals with the rotary force at the distal carpal row.
Care should be taken that the outrigger is centrally located so
that the wrist is flexed in a midline axis with slight ulnar deviation.
The base of the splint should not extend past the wrist flexion
crease, which would block palmar flexion.

ELBOW SPLINTS 9

STATIC ELBOW SPLINT

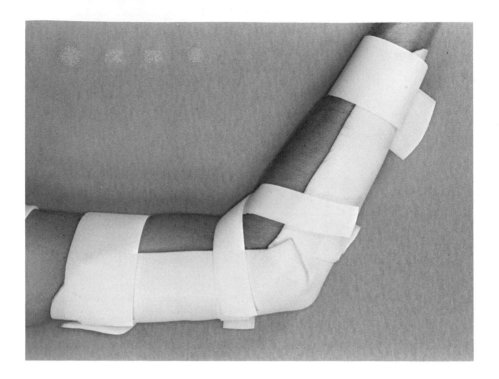

Type: Static

Purpose: This splint is worn to immobilize the elbow. When used in com-
                 bination with a wrist immobilization splint, it enables the fo-
                 rearm to be positioned in the neutral position, supination, or
                 pronation.

Indications: The splint is used postoperatively following:
                     Lateral epicondylectomy
                     Medial epicondylectomy
                     Cubital tunnel release
                     Elbow arthroplasty
                     Radial nerve repair, proximal to the elbow
                     Anterior transposition of the ulnar nerve
                     Darrach procedure (forearm positioned in supination post-
                     operatively)
                     Elbow flexion contracture releases (often fitted volarly and
                     increased serially into extension)

Wearing Time: The splint is worn between exercises and at night until 6 weeks.
                 With elbow flexion contractures, the splint is generally worn
                 between exercise sessions to place the elbow collateral ligaments
                 and joint capsule on maintained stretch.

With radial nerve repairs, the elbow is placed in extension and then brought into flexion 30° each week. This is done from the 3rd to 6th week postoperatively.

Precautions: Potential areas for compression include the:
Axilla
Ulnar nerve at the elbow
Radial nerve just proximal to the elbow

Correct Fit: The splint is generally fit dorsally during the postoperative phase in 90° of flexion.
The volar approach is used when attempting to serially increase elbow extension.
Be sure to provide padding over the olecranon.

TURNBUCKLE SPLINT

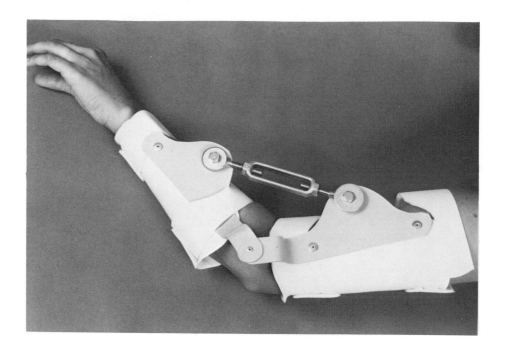

Type: Dynamic

Purpose: This splint is used to provide an adjustable dynamic force for elbow flexion or extension.

Indications: Limited elbow flexion or extension secondary to: trauma, immobilization, or following release of an elbow flexion contracture

Wearing Time: The splint is worn between exercises during the day; the patient wears a static elbow extension splint at night.

Precautions: Watch for pressure from the straps and shoulder pain from the weight of the splint.
Be especially watchful for potential compression of the radial nerve proximal to the elbow.

Correct Fit: The upper arm and forearm troughs should span two-thirds the length of both areas.
The turnbuckle should have enough length to allow full extension.
Typically, a 4- to 6-inch turnbuckle may be used; however, the size must be individually determined based on the size of the patient and degree of flexion contracture.

INNOVATIVE SPLINTS AND MOBILIZATION TECHNIQUES 10

DYNAMIC THUMB IP FLEXION SPLINT

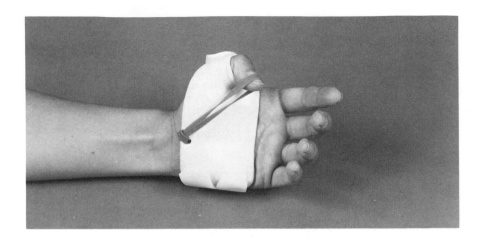

Type: Dynamic

Purpose: This splint may be used to obtain passive IP joint motion of the thumb. This is accomplished by dynamically assisting the IP joint into flexion without stressing the CMC and MP joints.

Indications: Conditions which may benefit from this splint include:
Arthrofibrosis of the IP joint of the thumb
Clinically healed fractures of the proximal or distal phalanx (6 to 8 weeks postoperatively)
EPL repair (a minimum of 6 weeks postoperatively)
Dorsal capsulotomies of the IP joint of the thumb

Wearing Time: The amount and length of wearing time will depend upon the severity of arthrofibrosis or capsular tightness. As a general rule, dynamic splints should not be worn for more than 1 hour without an associated exercise program.

Precautions: Pressure areas to be watchful of include:
The area just proximal to the IP flexion crease of the thumb and the distal palmar flexion crease of the index MP joint.

Correct Fit: The splint should be fitted as a web spacer with an extension over the MP joint dorsally, and across the palm volarly for adequate immobilization.
The distal edge should allow full IP motion without impingement.
A 90° angle of pull to the distal phalanx is essential.
The MP joint should be adequately immobilized to provide an effective dynamic pull on the distal phalanx.

BUDDY TAPES

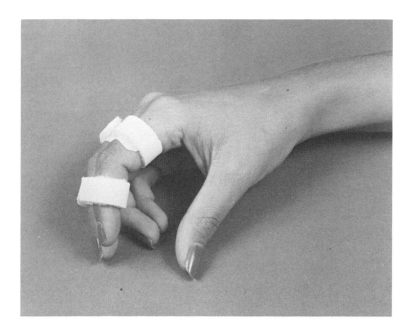

Type: Static

Purpose: These prefabricated devices may be used to secure one finger to an adjacent digit and allow full digital function.

Indications: Buddy tapes are used primarily:
To prevent ulnar or radial deviation of the PIP joint following PIP joint replacement arthroplasty
For strains of the radial or ulnar collateral ligaments of the MP or PIP joints
For exercise purposes, to use the ROM of a normal digit to assist a digit that does not have full function
To protect nondisplaced fractures of the proximal and middle phalanx and allow early ROM if:
the fracture is truly stable with no displacement in any plane and follow-up x-rays are taken to determine any developing displacement or angulation

Wearing Time: The buddy tapes are worn continuously except in those cases where they are used for exercise only.

Precautions: Buddy tapes should not be used on an edematous digit.

Correct Fit: Two tapes are used, each approximately ½" wide. The first is brought between the two digits to be taped, wrapped around the proximal phalanx of each digit and then secured back upon itself. The second tape is applied in the same manner around the middle phalanx.

ULNAR DRIFT SPLINT*

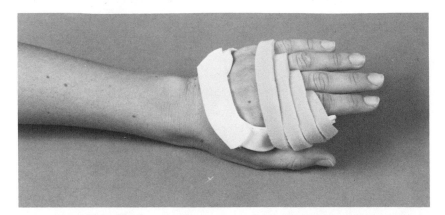

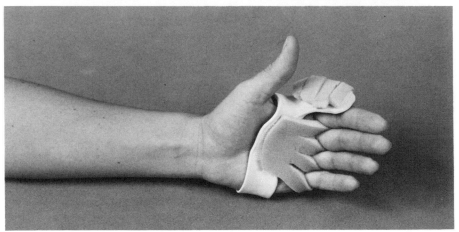

Type:	Static
Purpose:	This splint is used to support laterally the proximal phalanges of the index through small fingers in as close to neutral alignment as possible.
Indications:	Conservative management of rheumatoid arthritis to enhance functional use of the hand Following MP arthroplasties this splint may be worn to maintain proper digital alignment once the RA splint is discontinued.
Wearing Time:	The splint may be worn at all times during the day for improved comfort and function of the hand. It is important to perform

* This splint designed by Linwood J. Thomes, OTR, Lieutenant Colonel, Army Medical Specialist Corps, US Army; Assistant Chief Occupational Therapy Section Walter Reed Army Medical Center Washington, DC, and modified by the Hand Rehabilitation Center of Indiana, Inc.

passive ROM exercises with the digits each day to ensure the MP joints do not become stiff.

Precautions: The splint should allow full range of motion of the digits.
The development of pressure areas between the fingers and through the web spaces should be monitored.

Correct Fit: The volar support should rest along the transverse metacarpal arch in the palm.
There should be a lateral guard beside, but not touching, the second metacarpal head.
The straps should originate from the lateral guard and should be individually wrapped around the index, long, ring, and small fingers. They should then be brought back around dorsally and attached to the lateral guard.

BOWLING ALLEY SPLINT

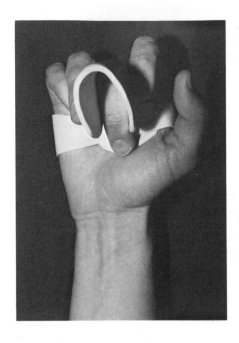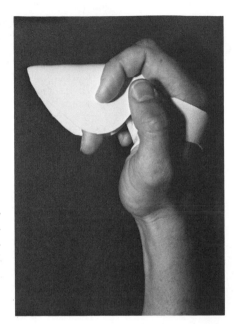

Type:	Static
Purpose:	To provide lateral support of the PIP and DIP joints when exercising
Indications:	This splint is used primarily to prevent lateral stress or deviation of the PIP joint while performing active and/or passive range-of-motion exercises. It is indicated following PIP joint replacement arthroplasty or reconstruction of the radial or ulnar collateral ligament of the PIP joint.
Wearing Time:	The splint is worn during exercise sessions only.
Precautions:	The lateral supports of the splint must not restrict range of motion of the digit.
Correct Fit:	The splint is made from a triangular piece of material which has approximately 4″ lateral supports. The base of the triangle is placed distal to the dorsal MP joint. The remaining two sides are then brought from the dorsum of the digit volarward to form the two lateral supports of the "alley." Care must be taken to ensure that there is enough room for full finger flexion and that no joint deviation is allowed within the splint.

MP DORSAL EXTENSION BLOCK

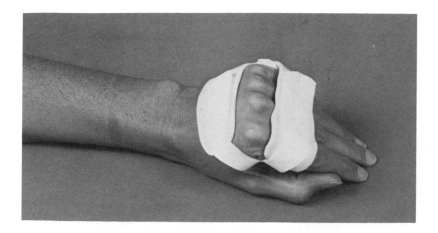

Type:
Static

Purpose:
The purpose of this splint is to prevent MP joint hyperextension, yet facilitate extension of the IP's and allow full flexion of the digits.

Indications:
This splint may be used for a combined median and ulnar nerve palsy where there is apparent clawing and a Wynn-Parry splint is not feasible. This is a good alternative splint for children.

Wearing Time:
The splint should be worn continuously for approximately 1 year to prevent the need for tendon transfers to correct the clawing deformity.

Precautions:
The MP joints need to be adequately secured by the splint so as not to allow hyperextension.
Pressure areas to watch include the skin along the transverse palmar arch, the dorsal surface of the proximal phalanx, and the first web space.

Correct Fit:
The splint is made from a rectangular piece of material approximately 3" × 2½". Two cuts are then made lengthwise to form a "W" with the center bar approximately ½" wide. The splint is then formed from the ulnar side of the hand. The center of the "W" forms a palmar bar, with the two remaining bars forming dorsal bands along the proximal phalanges, just proximal to the MP joints. The splint should hold the MP joints in approximately 45° of flexion at rest and prevent hyperextension upon active motion. It is then secured with a "Y"-shaped strap from the palmar bar, through the 1st web space and to each dorsal bar.

DIGITAL DORSAL EXTENSION BLOCK

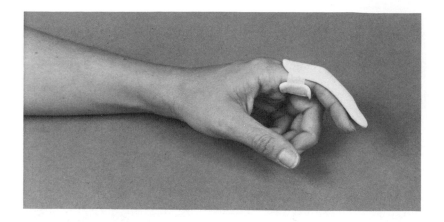

Type: Static

Purpose: The purpose of the splint is to prevent PIP extension to neutral, yet allow PIP and DIP joint flexion.

Indications: Conditions which may benefit from this splint include:
Swan neck deformity (for positioning *not* correction of the deformity)
Postoperatively following Littler lateral band tenodesis
Dorsal dislocations of the PIP joint
Postoperatively following digital nerve repairs

Wearing Time: When the splint is applied for the above indications, it is worn continuously with the appropriate exercises performed within the confines of the splint. Specific wearing periods include:
Swan neck deformity: as desired by the patient to improve functional use of the hand.
Littler lateral band tenodesis: continual wear until 6 to 8 weeks postoperatively. The splint may then be discontinued as long as hyperextension is not present.
Dorsal PIP joint dislocations and digital nerve repairs: the splint is worn continually for 6 weeks.

Precautions: The splint must not allow PIP extension beyond 30°.
The volar band around P_1 must not block PIP joint flexion.
Pressure areas to be watchful of include the dorsum of the PIP joint and the PIP flexion crease.

Correct Fit: The proximal bar must fit securely around the proximal phalanx to avoid extension of the PIP joint within the splint. The dorsal hood of the splint should hold the PIP joint in 30° of flexion.

SWAN NECK SPLINT

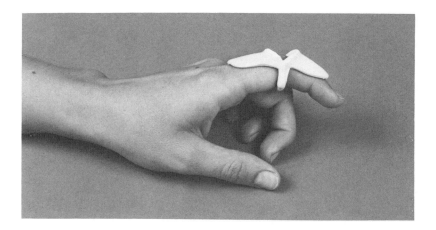

Type: Static

Purpose: This splint is used as a functional assist for flexible swan neck deformities to prevent PIP joint hyperextension.

Indications: It is primarily indicated as an assistive device for flexible swan neck deformities.

Wearing Time: The splint may be worn as needed as a functional assist.

Precautions: The splint must conform snugly about the PIP joint and yet allow for easy removal. This splint should not be used where edema is present or immediately postoperatively due to its circumferential nature.

Correct Fit: The splint is formed from a rectangular piece of material approximately 1" × 2", with two ⅛" holes drilled in the center, approximately ½" apart. The digit is pushed up through the proximal hole, and then down through the distal hole, forming a volar "bar" under the PIP joint and two dorsal "hoods" which hold the PIP joint in approximately 30° of flexion. It should allow full flexion of the PIP joint while preventing PIP joint hyperextension.

BOUTONNIÈRE SPLINT

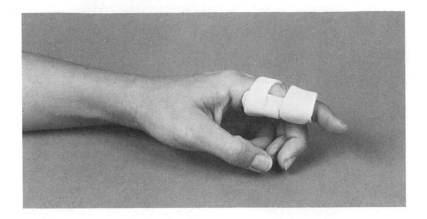

Type: Static

Purpose: This splint is primarily used following acute and chronic bou-
                    tonnière deformities to immobilize the PIP joint at neutral while
                    allowing full active and passive range-of-motion exercises to the
                    MP and DIP joint.

Indications: Acute or chronic boutonnière deformity
                    Following reconstructive procedures to the central slip (e.g., El-
                    liott repair)

Wearing Time: The splint is worn continually for 6 to 8 weeks before ROM
                    exercises are initiated. (Note: For chronic boutonniere deform-
                    ities, the PIP must be mobilized to 0° passively before this splint
                    may be utilized.)

Precautions: The PIP joint must be passively mobile to 0° of extension for
                    proper fitting of the splint.
                    The distal wrap-around band must not be constrictive.
                    The proximal edge of the splint must be sufficiently long to se-
                    cure the proximal phalanx.

Correct Fit: The splint is fit volarly holding the PIP joint in full extension
                    with a distal wrap-around band fit just proximal to the DIP flex-
                    ion crease.

VELCRO TRAPPERS

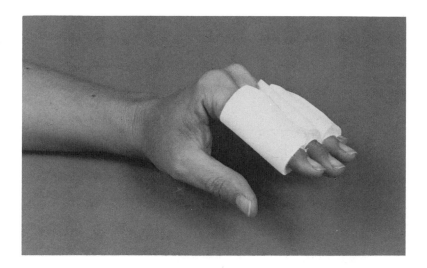

Type:	Treatment technique
Purpose:	These prefabricated devices may be used to assist in exercising the MP joints by eliminating or minimizing motion at the PIP and DIP joints. This allows all ROM to be concentrated at the MP joint level.
Indications:	These devices may be indicated whenever dorsal capsular tightness, arthrofibrosis, or limited motion is present at the MP joints.
Wearing Time:	Used for exercise sessions as an assistive device to increase active MP flexion
Precautions:	The Velcro may cause irritation to the dorsum of the PIP joints as the patient exercises.
Correct Fit:	The 2″ Velcro trappers are wrapped circumferentially around any two digits with the dividing seam between the digits. The patient exercises the MP joints while wearing the trappers.

FINGER TAPING

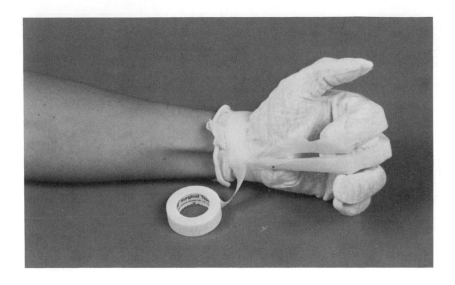

Type: Mobilization technique

Purpose: Taping is primarily used to increase passive MP, PIP, and DIP joint motion of the hand and/or aid in resolving extrinsic extensor tightness.

Indications: Dorsal capsular tightness or arthrofibrosis of the MP, PIP, and/or DIP joints of the hand.
Extrinsic extensor tightness

Wearing Time: The tape is left on for a full 20-minute session during which time additional layers of tape may be added to bring the joints into increased flexion serially. In the case of extrinsic extensor tightness, a 1 or 2 lb weight may be added to the dorsum of the hand to passively stretch the wrist into increased flexion.

Precautions: Digits with severe edema or compromised circulation should not be taped.
Circumferential taping is contraindicated with PIP joint arthroplasties.

Correct Fit: A lightweight cotton glove is placed over the hand.
The proximal edge of the glove is secured with a piece of 1" tape around the wrist.
½" tape is placed circumferentially around the PIP and DIP joints of each digit bringing them into as much passive flexion as possible.
Tape is then brought from the dorsum of the wrist, over each digit and secured to the volar wrist. Each digit is taped in this fashion to bring them into flexion.
Additional layers are added as tolerated to bring the digits into further flexion serially.

THUMB TAPING

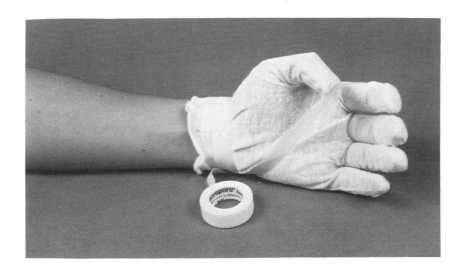

Type:	Mobilization technique
Purpose:	Taping is primarily used to increase passive MP and IP joint motion of the thumb.
Indications:	Dorsal capsular tightness or arthrofibrosis of the MP and/or IP joints of the thumb Extrinsic extensor tightness of the EPL
Wearing Time:	The tape is left on for a full 20-minute session during which time additional layers of tape may be added to serially bring the joints into increased flexion. In the case of extrinsic extensor tightness, a 1 or 2 lb weight may be added to the dorsum of the hand to passively stretch the wrist.
Precautions:	Taping should not be performed on digits with severe edema or in the presence of compromised circulation.
Correct Fit:	A lightweight cotton glove is placed over the hand. The proximal edge of the glove is secured with a piece of 1″ tape around the wrist. ½″ tape is placed from the proximal wrist, brought along the dorsum of the thumb, down to the ulnar side of the wrist and secured, thereby bringing the thumb into flexion. Additional layers are added as tolerated to bring the thumb into further flexion serially.

COBAN TAPING

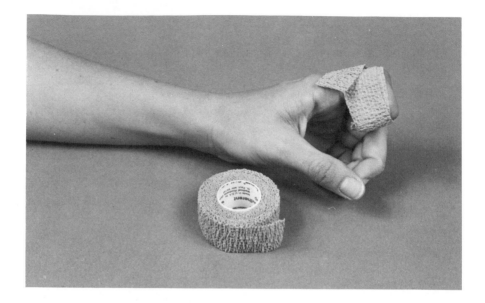

Type:	Mobilization technique
Purpose:	Taping is primarily used to increase passive PIP and DIP joint motion.
Indications:	Dorsal capsular tightness or arthrofibrosis of the PIP and/or DIP joints of the digits Intrinsic tightness
Wearing Times:	The Coban tape is left on for a 10- to 20-minute session during which time additional layers of Coban tape may be added to bring the joints into increased flexion serially.
Precautions:	Taping should not be performed on digits with severe edema or compromised circulation. Circumferential taping is contraindicated with PIP and DIP joint arthroplasties.
Correct Fit:	A ½″ piece of Coban tape approximately 12 inches long is placed circumferentially around the PIP and DIP joints of the affected digit, bringing them into as much passive flexion as possible. The tape may be tightened or additional layers added as tolerated to bring the digits into further flexion serially. If Coban taping is done with patients with mild intrinsic tightness the patient must exercise the MP in extension once the tape has been applied.

GLOVE RUBBER BANDS (GRB's)

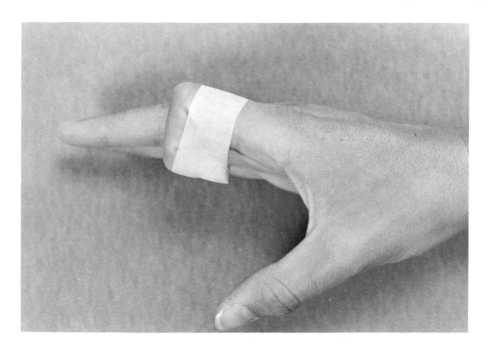

Type:	Treatment technique
Purpose:	To increase passive PIP and/or DIP flexion
Indications:	Dorsal capsular tightness of the PIP and/or DIP joints
Wearing Times:	GRB's are worn for a maximum of 5- to 10-minute sessions.
Precautions:	Watch for vascular compromise Should not be used with: Edematous digits PIP/DIP arthroplasties Ring avulsion injuries Vascular disorders (i.e., raynauds' phenomenon, systemic lupus erythematosus, scleroderma)
Correct Fit:	The digit is held in as much flexion as possible. The glove rubber band is then placed on the distal phalanx and brought around the proximal phalanx as shown. (Note: Glove rubber bands are cut from the digital portion of Pharmaseal surgical gloves. The cut segments are approximately ½″ wide.)

WIDE RUBBER BANDS (WRB's)

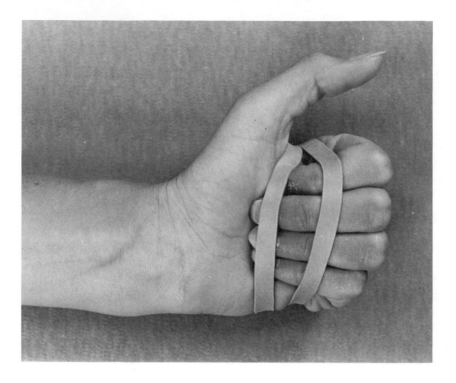

Type:	Treatment technique
Purpose:	To increase passive PIP and/or DIP flexion
Indications:	Limited passive flexion of the PIP and/or DIP joints secondary to extensor tendon or dorsal capsular tightness
Wearing Times:	The rubber bands should be worn for a maximum of 10-minute sessions.
Precautions:	Watch for vascular compromise WRB's are contraindicated when edema is present and with PIP/DIP arthroplasties.
Correct Fit:	The wide rubber band should be applied over the dorsum of the metacarpals and then over P_2 and/or P_3 as indicated. (Note: #73 pure rubber bands are used.)

BIBLIOGRAPHY

1. A.A.O.S.: Atlas of Orthotics, Biomechanical Principles and Applications. CV Mosby Co., St. Louis, 1975

2. Bunch WT, Keagy RD: Principles of Orthotic Treatment. CV Mosby Co., St. Louis, 1976

3. Calliet R: Hand Pain and Impairment, 2nd Ed. FA Davis Co., Philadelphia, 1976

4. Fess E, Gettle K, Strickland JW: Hand Splinting Principles and Methods. CV Mosby Co., St. Louis, 1982

5. Green DP, McCoy H: Turnbuckle orthotic correction of elbow-flexion contractures after acute injuries. J Bone Joint Surg (A) 61:1092–1095, 1979

6. Hunter JM, Schneider LH, Mackin EJ, Bell JA: Rehabilitation of the Hand. CV Mosby Co., St. Louis, 1978

7. Melvin JL: Rheumatic Disease: Occupational Therapy and Rehabilitation. FA Davis Co., Philadelphia, 1977

8. Wolfort FG: Acute Hand Injuries. Little, Brown and Co., Boston, 1980

9. Wynn-Parry CB: Rehabilitation of the Hand, 4th Ed. Butterworths, London, 1981